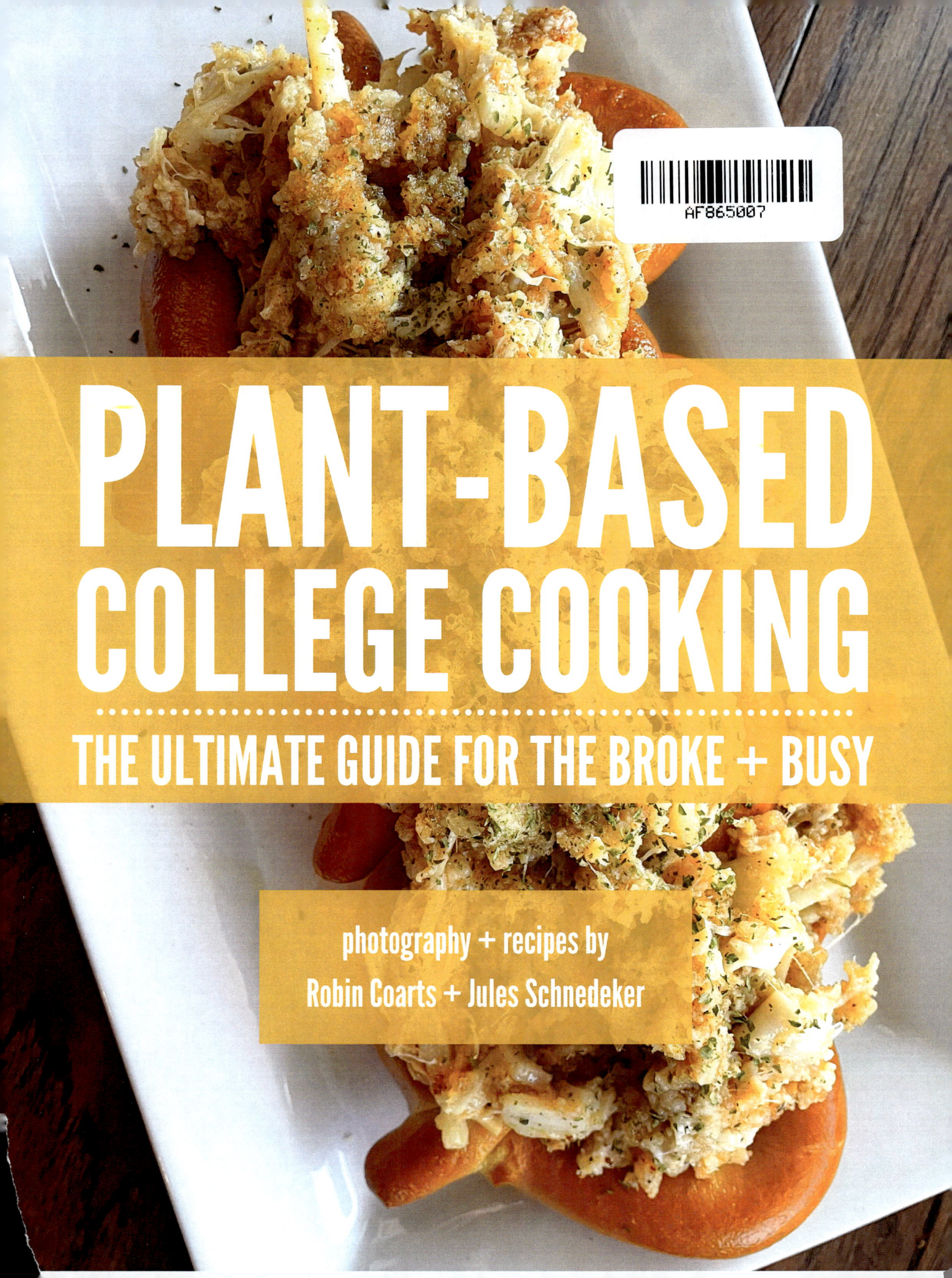

PLANT-BASED COLLEGE COOKING

THE ULTIMATE GUIDE FOR THE BROKE + BUSY

photography + recipes by
Robin Coarts + Jules Schnedeker

PLANT-BASED COLLEGE COOKING:
The Ultimate Guide for the Broke + Busy

Published by:
Plant-Based Point
70 SW Century Dr
Ste 100 PMB 5001
Bend, OR 97702

ISBN: 978-1-7370650-2-9 (print)
978-1-7370650-1-2 (eBook)

Design + photography
by
Robin Coarts + Jules Schnedeker

1st Edition, 2022

For more information, please visit: https://plantbasedpoint.com.

this book is dedicated to

those whose idea of success is spelled with

love and compassion

for all living beings

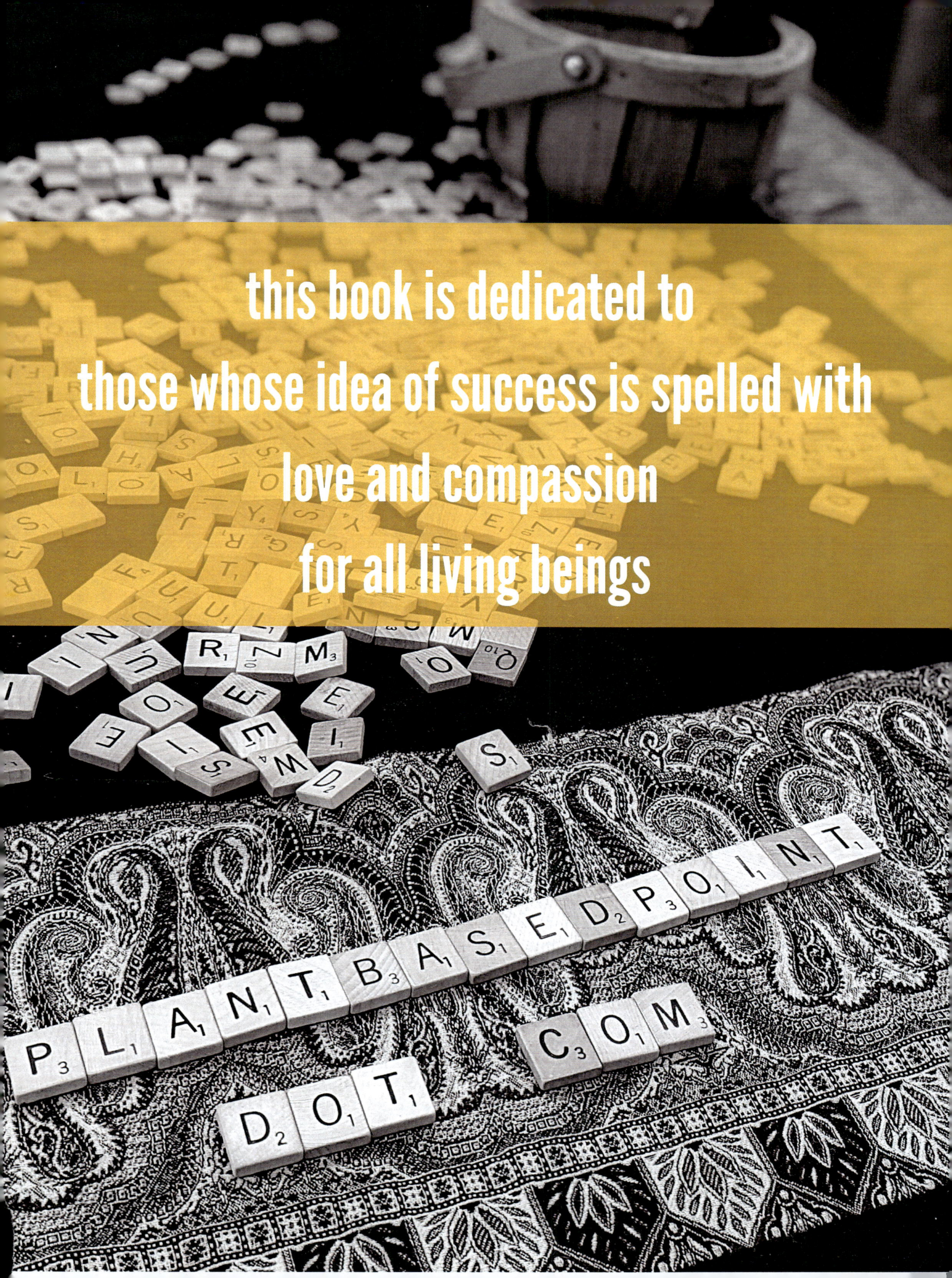

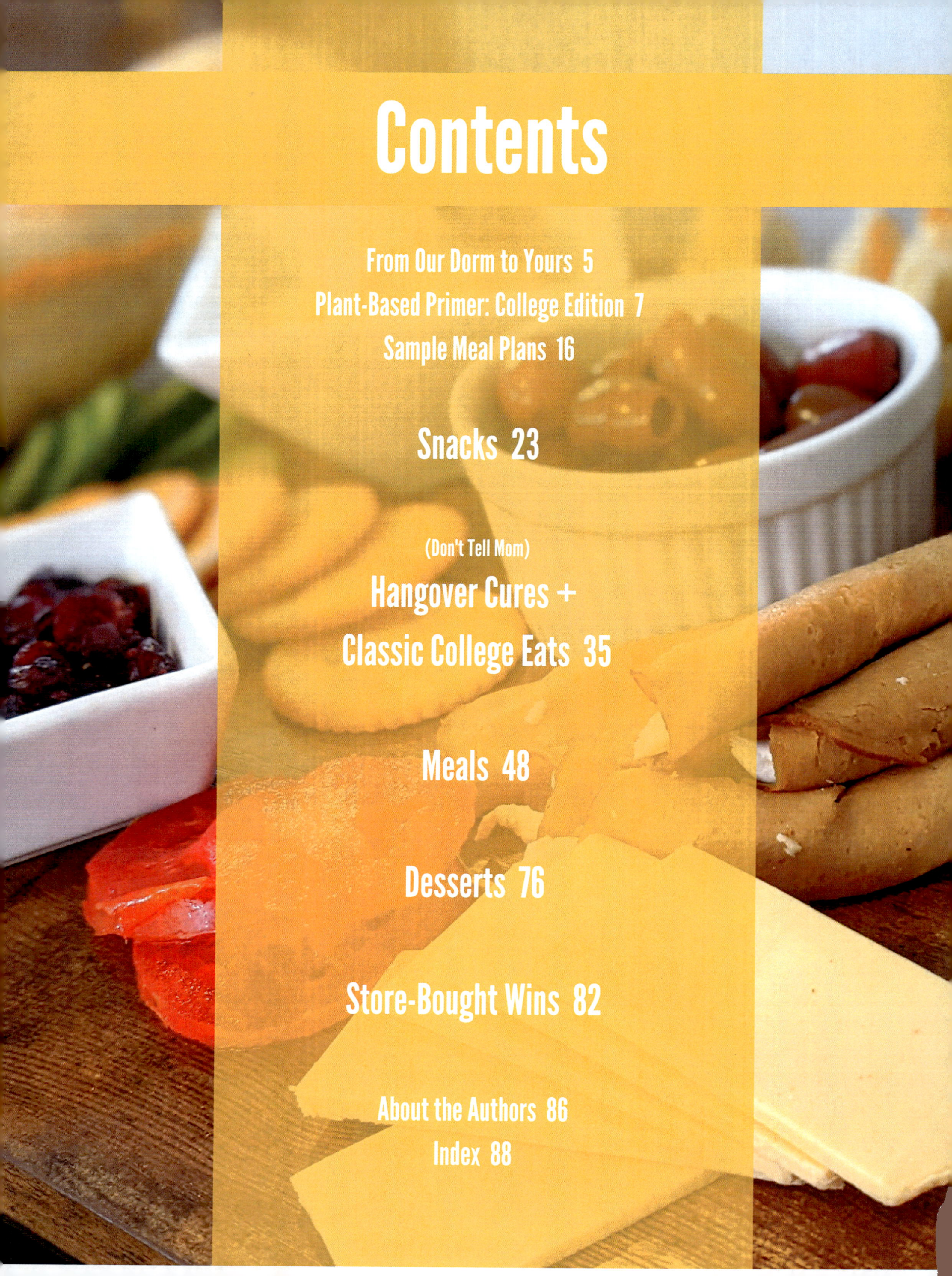

Contents

From Our Dorm to Yours

Hey, Smarty Pants!

We heard you had brains, and now that you're reading this, we know it's true. You're probably bouncing between classes right now, so we'll make this quick. Thanks for grabbing this guide that's sure to satisfy any craving without breaking the bank.

We recommend taking a quick peek at the primer, then follow your taste buds as you peruse the table of contents! An easy way to save money during your weekly grocery run: find a few recipes that use the same ingredients so you can cross-purpose them, e.g., potatoes, peanut butter, or beans. (Bonus: most of these will keep for a while, too!)

Share With Us

We love seeing your kitchen handiwork. Tag @plantbasedpoint across social media to share your creations!

Questions? Let us know! You can also find recipe videos and cooking tutorials on our YouTube channel (@plantbasedpoint). Happy cooking!

Sincerely,
robin + jules
proud founders of
PLANT-BASED POINT

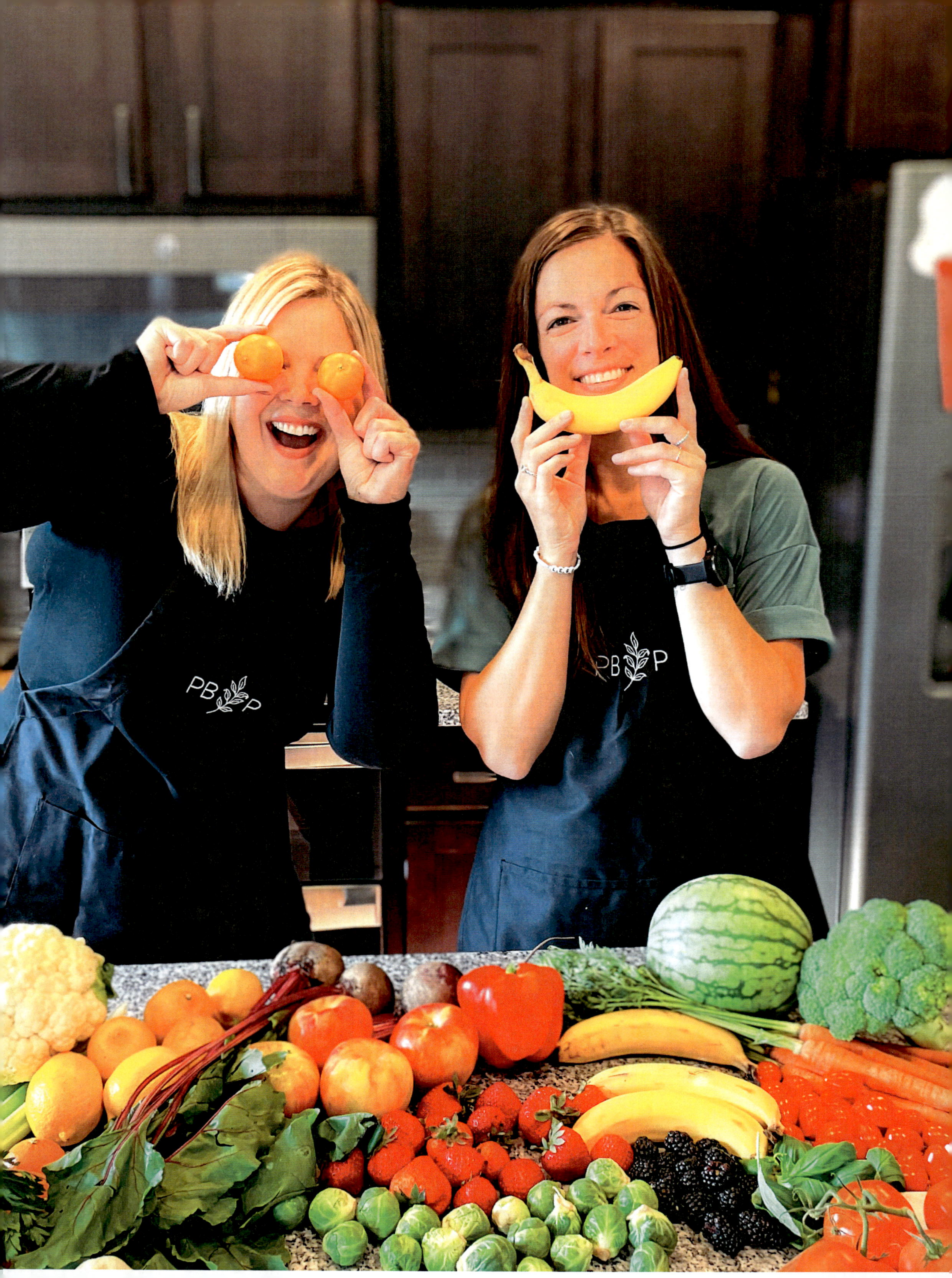
PBP
PBP

Plant-Based Primer College Edition

New to plant-based eating? Here's a little starter kit to get you going, and you can find even more tips and tools on our website, including a free, printable, plant-based primer: PlantBasedPoint.com.

On the 'Our Favorite Products' page of our website, we include a lot of our top products and brands. With all of the new plant-based items consistently hitting the shelves, this is an ever-evolving list! Here are a few things that never change:

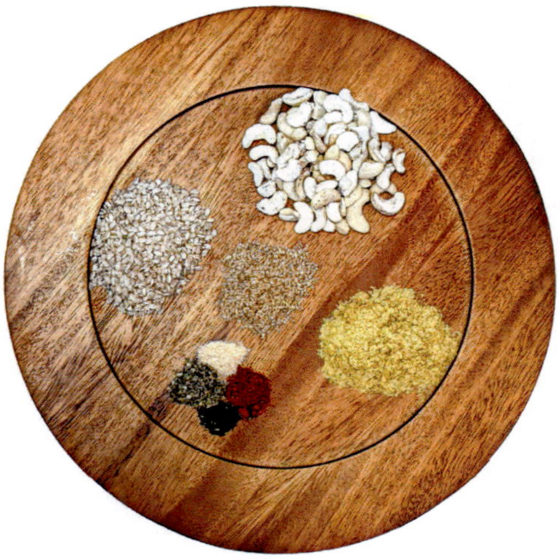

Cheap pantry staples

- Agave
- Coconut milk
- Dried beans (especially chickpeas, mung beans, black beans)
- Grains (brown rice, quinoa, bulger)
- Nutritional yeast (gives your dishes a salty, cheesy-like taste that you'll grow to love if you don't already)
- Peanut butter
- Spices (especially smoked paprika, garlic powder, dill, oregano)
- Tahini
- Unsweetened plant-based milk
- Vegetable broth

Substitutions + Swaps

Oil or vegan butter	Water or vegetable broth. For baked goods, you can use applesauce
Nuts	Many nuts are interchangeable or can be substituted with shelled sunflower seeds or pepitas (shelled pumpkin seeds)
Soy	You can easily swap tofu or tempeh with beans or plant-based meat
Gluten	Feel free to use gluten-free flours, pie crusts, breadcrumbs, and pastry, etc.
Onions TOP TIP!	You can get the rich, savory taste of onions on the cheap -and without cooking- by buying a bunch of scallions (green onions) for about a dollar, rinsing, and snipping into bite-sized pieces with clean scissors!
Fresh vs. dried herbs	Generally 1 teaspoon dried = 1 tablespoon fresh

To make the recipes in this cookbook...

...you will need:

- Microwave
- Mini fridge
- Hot plate (or stovetop) - for select recipes
- Toaster oven - for select recipes
- Can opener
- Pot with lid
- Large spoon to stir
- Standard plates/bowls/utensils (to chow down)
- Microwave safe containers (to store leftovers and microwave dishes)
- Sharp knife

...you won't need:

- Blender
- Food processor
- Pressure cooker
- Full-sized oven
- Fancy kitchen utensils
- A fat wallet

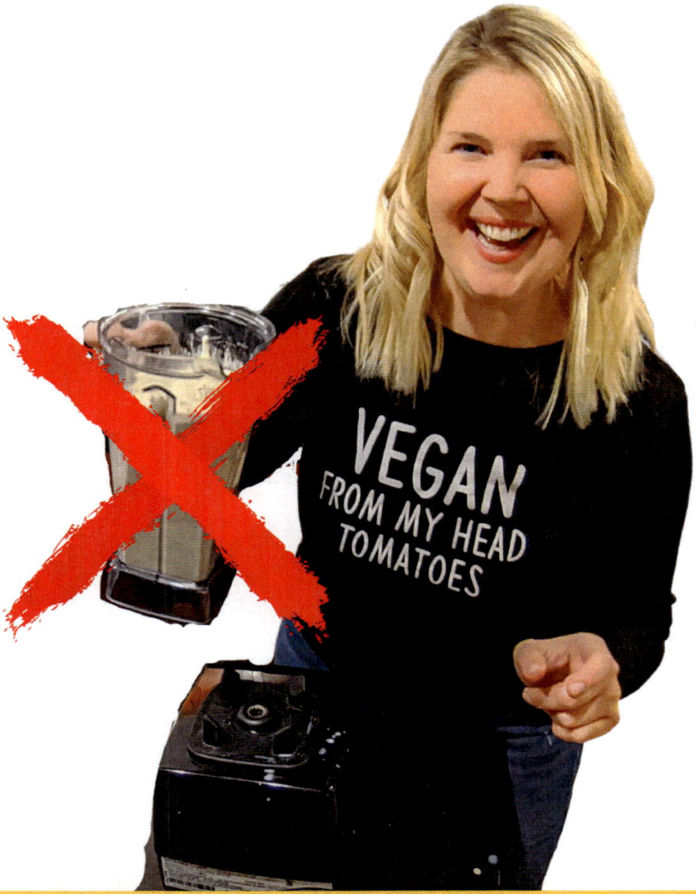

Notes

STORAGE

We didn't include storage instructions for each recipe as they all follow the same general rule: Store refrigerated, in an airtight container, for up to 5-7 days.

SERVING SIZES

We designed this guidebook for the busy individual who wants to whip up a quick meal for one (or two). All recipes can easily be doubled, tripled, etc. if you're feeding more or want to batch cook and have extra meals throughout the hectic week.

MEASUREMENTS

Most measurements in this book are flexible and can be adjusted to suit your personal taste. Do you like more (or less) hummus, vegan mayo, etc.? Extra scallions and hot sauce? Go for it!

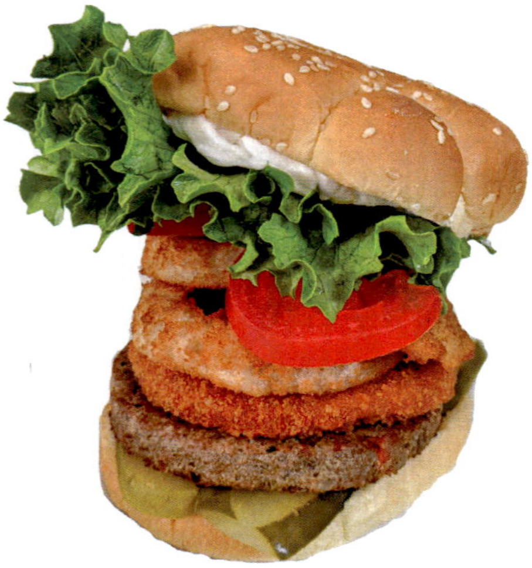

=

serving size one [hungry student]

Don't strain yourself...

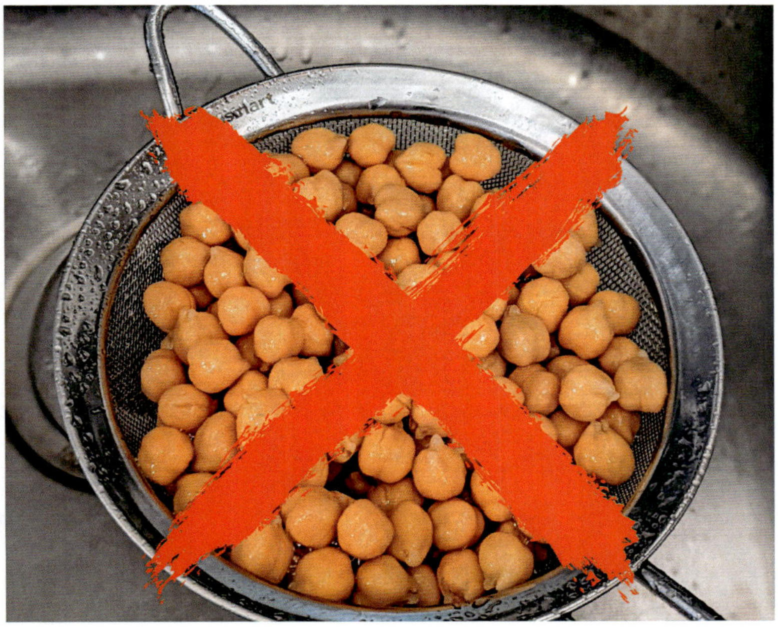

We designed this guidebook for those who might not have access to standard kitchen utensils. To strain or rinse rice, beans, or pasta, you can simply use the cooking pot and lid or the can that the item came in.

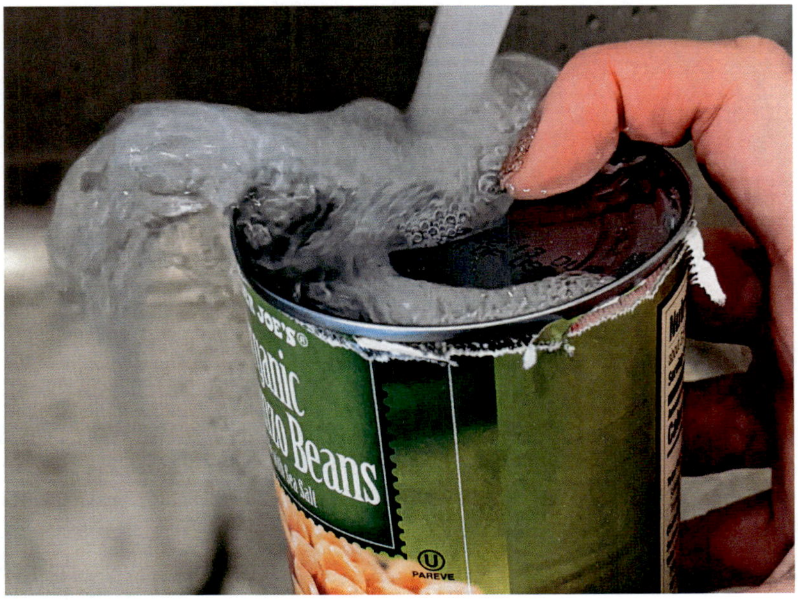

Accidentally Vegan (Mostly)

Throughout this guidebook, we mention ingredients that are accidentally vegan - USUALLY. Sometimes milk, eggs, and/or honey are hidden in the most surprising places, so be sure to check labels before buying.

This guidance applies to the following ingredients mentioned in this book:

- BBQ sauce
- Bread (rolls, sliced bread, tortillas)
- Crackers
- Dairy-free chocolate chips/chocolate candy
- Pasta
- Polenta (corn grits)
- Popcorn (microwavable)
- Pretzels (frozen)
- Vegetarian chili
- Vegetarian gravy
- Vegetarian refried beans

TIP: Jump to the bolded allergens section at the end of each ingredient label to see if the product contains milk, fish, or eggs.

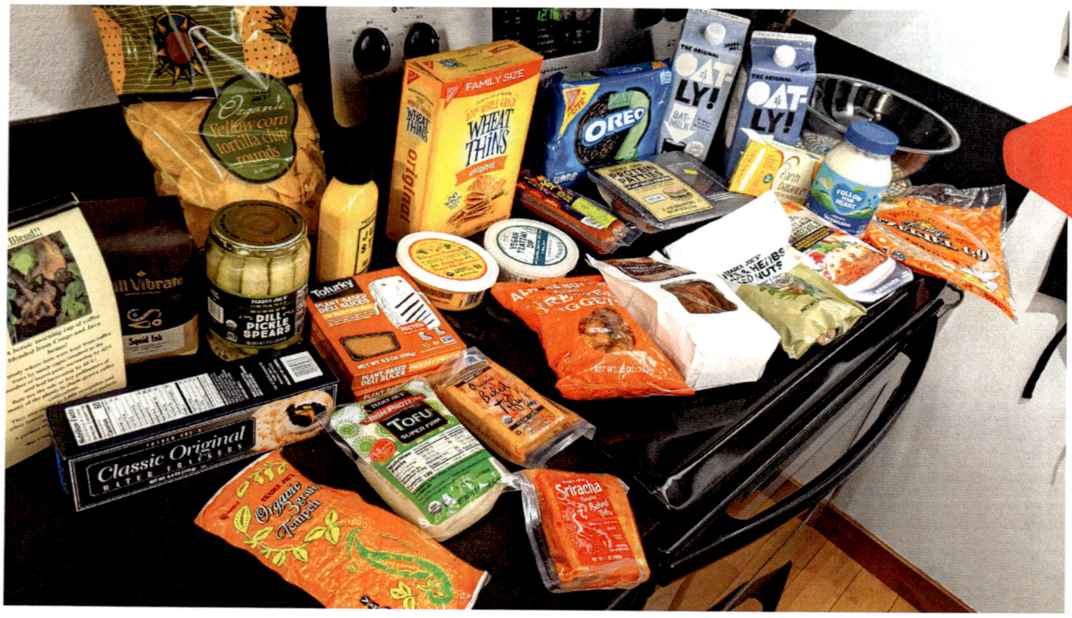

all accidentally vegan!

Why Vegan?

Whether you're interested in improving your health, the health of the planet, or the health of our non-human animal friends, eating a plant-based diet is one of the easiest -and most fun!- ways you can achieve that goal.

Eating a plant-based diet can...

- reduce inflammation (are you a college athlete or training for a race? Plant-based foods can speed up recovery time!)
- increase energy
- lower "bad" cholesterol
- increase fiber intake
- reduce your chances of diabetes, osteoporosis, and heart disease
- save 105 animals per year[1]
- save 620 pounds of harmful carbon dioxide emissions, 913 square feet of forest, and 33,481 gallons of water per month[2]

For more in-depth guidance, check out the Resources page on our website!

A note about protein

Generally speaking, as long as you're consuming enough calories, you're getting enough protein. And while almost no one is protein-deficient, 95% of Americans ARE fiber-deficient. Which brings us to...

Did you know...?

Cholesterol is only found in animal products and fiber is only found in plant-based food. VEGAN WIN!

[1] https://plantbasednews.org/culture/ethics/105-animals-saved-a-year-by-eating-plant-based-study-finds/
[2] https://www.veestro.com/blogs/food-for-thought/what-difference-can-one-person-make-by-going-vegan

"Vegan" vs. "Plant-Based"

Vegan = Belief System

While often used interchangeably with "plant-based," the term "vegan" actually applies to an entire belief system. If a person identifies as vegan, it means that they believe non-human animals should not be used for human benefit. There are a lot of gray areas, but generally speaking, a vegan abstains from any activity in which an animal is exploited for profit (zoos, aquariums, horseback riding, etc.) and does not eat, wear, or use any product containing animal products or that has been tested on animals.

An "ethical vegan" is someone who chooses a vegan lifestyle primarily because of this belief system, and not for their own health. Many people start with a vegan diet for health reasons and, over time (as they learn more about animal explotation), adopt this ethical stance.

Plant-Based = Diet

The term "plant-based" refers strictly to the food one consumes (i.e., their diet). Many people who eat a plant-based, or primary plant-based, diet do not identify as vegan or subscribe to that belief system.

A word of caution: Check your labels. Thanks to "green washing," some food and household items labeled "plant-based" still contain animal products or have been tested on animals.

Neither "vegan" nor "plant-based" should be considered synonymous with "healthy" or "safe." If health is your top concern, consider...

Whole Food(s) Plant Based

This term refers to plant-based foods eaten in their most natural, unprocessed form. If health is your top priority, you might want to consider a "whole food(s) plant-based" diet.

money-saving tips

- Create a weekly meal plan (see next section) and try to use the same ingredients in multiple meals, e.g., potatoes, peanut butter, or beans. (Bonus: most of these will keep for a while, too!)
- Buy one fresh herb (usually very inexpensive) for the week that you can use to punch up a bunch of recipes, e.g., scallions, parsley, cilantro, etc. - gourmet-style on the cheap! (And looks great for those social media food pics.)

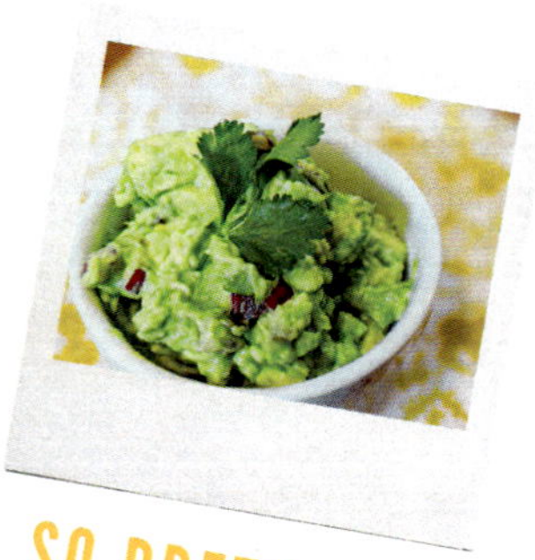

SO PRETTY...

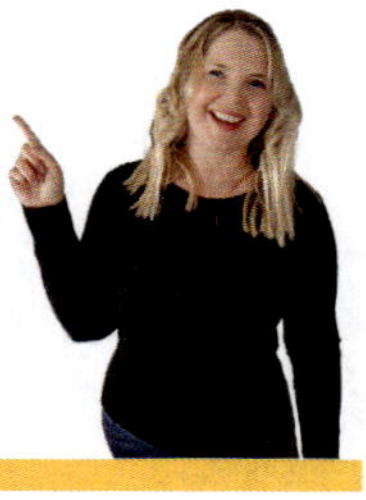

JULES'S TOP TIP

When trying any new plant-based recipes, food items, or products, think of it like switching from an old favorite brand to a new one, e.g., Heinz to Hunts ketchup. The flavor (and maybe texture) might seem REALLY different - because your tastebuds just aren't used to it. **Yet**. But that doesn't mean it's bad! I hated nutritional yeast at first. Now? I can't live without it.

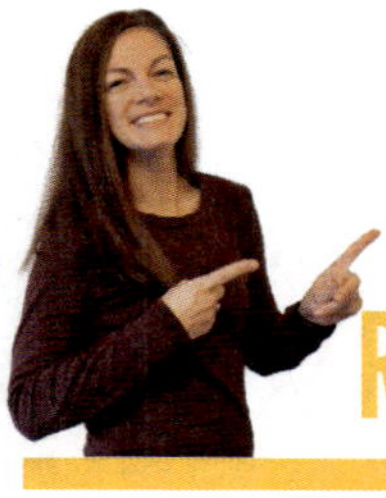

ROBIN'S TOP TIP

Read recipes before you begin, mark off your likes/dislikes, and dive in. If you don't like onions, skip 'em! If you love beans, double 'em! Don't be afraid to adjust recipes to your preferences. While you're learning recipes, figure out which kitchen tools you *must* have and which ones you can do without. Create a space that works for you and what you're cooking up.

SAMPLE MEAL PLANS

You're about to read one of the most valuable features of this guidebook: our sample meal plans and shopping lists!

Each of these weekly plans costs under $25 (at the time of publication) and will hopefully illustrate how to regularly create meal plans on a budget.

They are intended to be followed sequentially.

Follow us @plantbasedpoint for ongoing money-saving ideas and tips!

How to Meal Plan
(and how to use our meal plans)

- STEP 1: Think about the foods and flavors you most want to eat this week and jot them down. Try thinking about them in terms of a base and a theme, e.g., grains, lettuce, bread, tortillas, etc. + Asian, Italian, Indian, Thai, etc.
- STEP 2: Narrow down your list to a few dishes that share the most common ingredients and leverage pantry staples and spices you already have.
- STEP 3: Make your shopping list and get to the store!
- STEP 4 (optional): Once home from shopping, chop/wash/prep/store your items (or batch cook) for easy use throughout the week.

Using Our Meal Plans

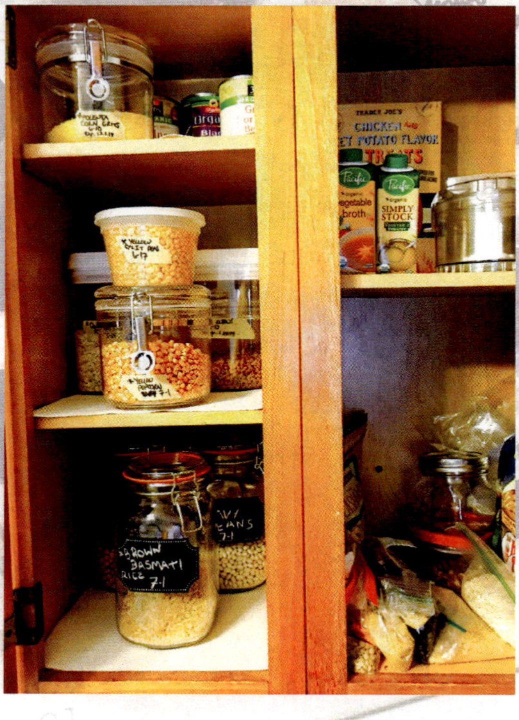

The following sample meal plans are meant to be followed sequentially to illustrate how you can build on pantry items that you only need to purchase once.

For example, in week one, you'll purchase sriracha and nutritional yeast and have plenty leftover for future weeks.

Each week will provide 10-20 individual meals, meant to be supplemented by cafeteria visits and outings with friends!

Shopping at bargain stores (e.g., Aldi, Trader Joe's) and in bulk will help keep costs down. If you have wiggle room in your weekly budget, we recommend buying extra fruits and veggies!

SAMPLE MEAL PLAN: WEEK #1

meals:

- Cheater Guacamole x 3* (page 26)
- Hash Brown Burrito x 4-5 (page 40)
- Loaded Sweet Potato x 3 (page 62)
- Quick Quesadilla x 4-5 (page 72)

*x 3 equals the number of times you can make this recipe based on your grocery list, e.g., for Week #1, you make 3 portions of the Cheater Guacamole recipe

This meal plan uses avocado, tortillas, vegan cheese, beans, sweet potatoes, greens, and hash browns across several dishes.

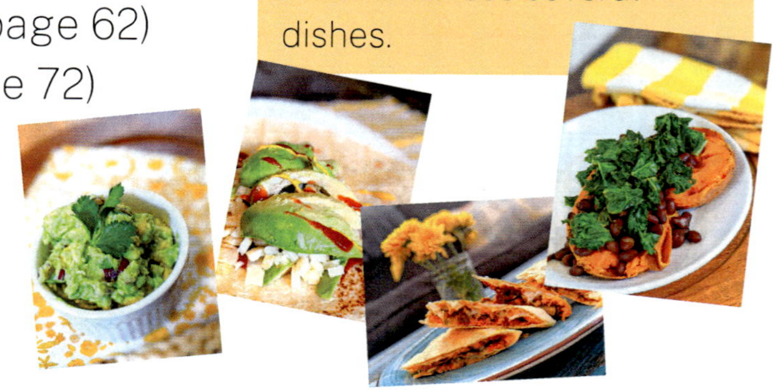

grocery list:

PREPARED:

- Black beans (2 15-oz cans)
- Salt (if needed)
- Sriracha or your favorite hot sauce (1 bottle)
- Tortillas (burrito-sized, 8 or 10-count pkg)
- Yellow mustard (optional)

FROZEN:

- Hash browns (1 30-oz pkg)

REFRIGERATED:

- Shredded vegan cheese of choice (1 pkg)

PRODUCE:

- Avocados (3)
- Greens (collards, kale, or spinach), 2 large bags
- Scallions (1 bunch)
- Sweet potatoes (1 2 or 3-lb bag)
- Red onion (1)

OTHER:

- Nutritional yeast (buy about 1 cup in bulk if possible)

notes:

- Use Cheater Guacamole alongside or in any of the other dishes
- Batch cook the entire bag of sweet potatoes and use in all recipes except Cheater Guacamole
- Leverage potatoes, beans, cheese, greens, red onion, scallions, nutritional yeast, and sriracha across all meals

SAMPLE MEAL PLAN: WEEK #2

meals:

This meal plan uses BBQ sauce, chickpeas, bread, and pickles across several meals and allows you to stock up on staples for future weeks.

- BBQ Chickpea Salad Boats x 2 (page 50)
- Oatmeal Bowls x 3-4 (page 64)
- Peanut Butter + Pickle Sandwich x 4-5 (page 46)
- Potato Chip Sandwich x 4-5 (page 47)

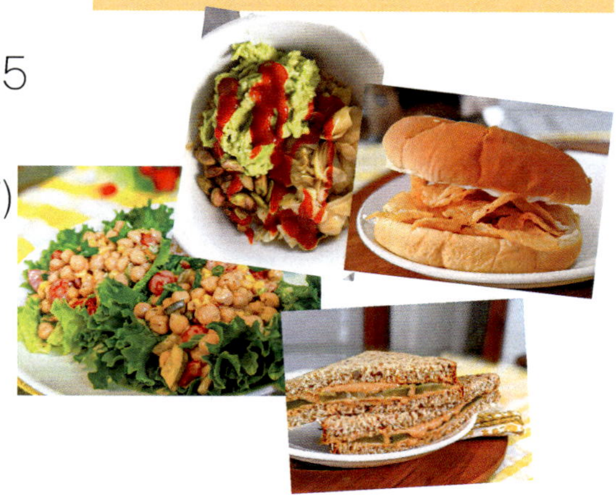

grocery list:

PREPARED:

- BBQ sauce (1 bottle)
- Bread (1 loaf)
- Chickpeas (2 15-oz cans)
- Peanut butter (1 jar)
- Pickle slices (1 jar - sweet or dill)
- Potato chips (1 8+ oz bag)
- Rolled oats (1 18-oz container or ~4 cups in bulk)
- Vegan mayo (1 jar)

FROZEN:

- Corn (1 bag)

PRODUCE:

- Avocado (1)
- Lettuce (romaine, green, or red) - 1 bunch or bag
- Scallions (1 bunch)
- Tomatoes (2)

notes:

- Make the BBQ Salad version of the Oatmeal Bowl and use BBQ sauce in both (BBQ sauce is also yummy mixed with mayo for the Potato Chip Sandwich!)
- Use pickles in Chickpea Salad and Peanut Butter + Pickle Sandwiches
- Use produce across recipes
- If you please, use the sriracha and yellow mustard you purchased last week on any of Week 2's meals!

SAMPLE MEAL PLAN: WEEK #3

meals:

- Cheater Peanut Sauce Pasta (page 54)
- Creamy Pumpkin Soup (page 56)
- Radical Rice + Beans (page 74)
- No Frills Chocolate Fondue (page 80)

This meal plan uses coconut cream across several meals and allows you to stock up on staples for future weeks.

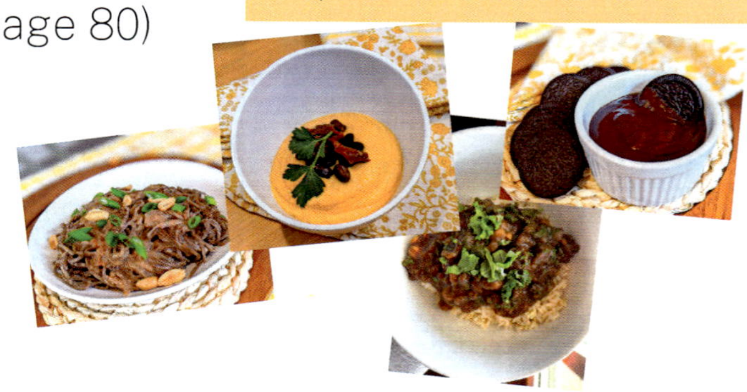

grocery list:

PREPARED:

- Agave (1 bottle)
- Black beans or black bean soup (1 15-oz can)
- Coconut cream (1 can)
- Noodles (angel hair, soba, or rice) - 1 pkg
- Pumpkin (1 15-oz can)
- Rice (any variety), 1 2-lb bag or buy in bulk
- Soy sauce (1 bottle)

PRODUCE:

- Bell pepper (green) - 1
- Greens (collards, kale, spinach) - 1 bunch or bag
- Scallions - 1 bunch

OTHER:

- Non-dairy chocolate chips (1 bag)
- Peanuts (buy 1+ cup in bulk if you can)
- Vegan cookies (Oreos, Nutter Butters, etc.) - 1 pkg

notes:

- Divvy up coconut cream as follows: All in Creamy Pumpkin Soup EXCEPT 2-3 TBSP reserved for No Frills Chocolate Fondue
- Leverage produce across recipes
- Feel free to make extra rice to enjoy with Cheater Peanut Sauce or Creamy Pumpkin Soup
- PANTRY STAPLES FROM PRIOR WEEKS TO USE: Nutritional yeast, peanut butter, sriracha

SAMPLE MEAL PLAN: WEEK #4

meals:

- Cheater Enchiladas (page 52)
- Creamy Tomato Soup + Rice (page 57)
- Hash Brown Burrito x 4-5 (page 40)
- Overnight Oats x 3-5 (page 65)

This meal plan uses tortillas, rice, and produce across several meals and gets your spice rack stocked.

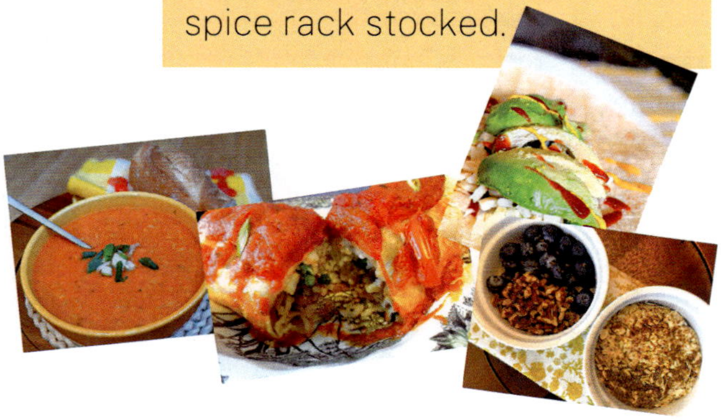

grocery list:

PREPARED:

- Black beans (2 15-oz cans)
- Burrito-sized tortillas (1 8 or 10-count pkg)
- Coconut milk (1 unsweetened, full fat, 15-ounce can)
- Tomato sauce (2 15-ounce cans, or 1 large 30+ ounce can)

REFRIGERATED:

- Non-dairy milk (1 container)
- Vegan pepperjack or cheddar cheese shreds (1 pkg)

PRODUCE:

- Avocados (2)
- Berries or Bananas (for Overnight Oats)
- Scallions (1 bunch)

OTHER:

- Cinnamon (optional)
- Garlic powder
- Onion powder
- Oregano

notes:

- Use hash browns (frozen; leftover from Week #1) and beans in both Cheater Enchiladas and Hash Brown Burritos
- PANTRY STAPLES FROM PRIOR WEEKS TO USE: Agave, frozen corn, frozen hash browns, mustard, nutritional yeast, oats, peanut butter, peanuts, rice, sriracha

SAMPLE MEAL PLAN: WEEK #5

meals:

This meal plan uses hummus and produce across meals and leverages plenty of pantry staples!

- Dessert Cups (page 78)
- Elevated Ramen x 3-4 (page 58)
- Panini Paradise x 4-5 (page 66)
- Salad Sandwich x 4-5 (page 75)

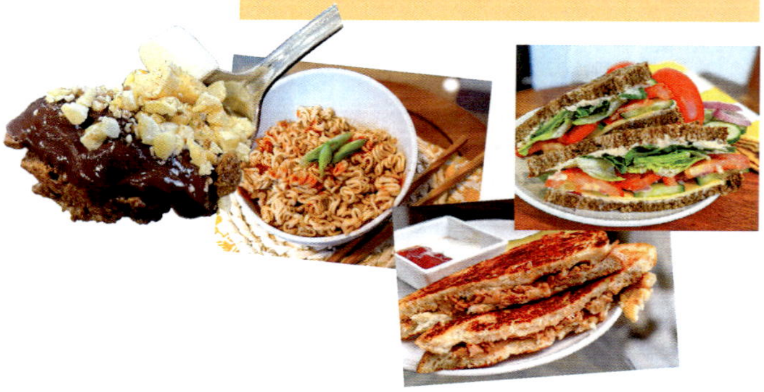

grocery list:

PREPARED:

- Bread (1 loaf)
- Ramen noodles (3-4 pkgs) - OR- 1-lb package other preferred pasta
- Rice vinegar (1 bottle)
- Vegan marshmallows (1 pkg)

REFRIGERATED:

- Hummus (2 small or 1 large container)
- Vegan cheese slices (1 pkg)
- Vegan butter (1 13-oz container or 2+ sticks)

PRODUCE:

- Cucumber (1)
- Spinach (1 bag)
- Red onion (1)
- Scallions (1 bunch)
- Tomatoes (3-4)

OTHER:

- Ginger Powder

notes:

- Use hummus, vegan cheese, and fresh produce in both Panini Paradise and Salad Sandwiches
- Make S'Mores option of Dessert Cups (using leftovers from prior weeks)
- Have leftover pickles or mustard? Use them in this week's sandwiches/paninis!
- PANTRY STAPLES TO USE FROM PRIOR WEEKS: agave, chocolate chips, ginger powder, peanut butter, soy sauce, sriracha, vegan cookies

Snacks

Charcuterie on the Cheap

serves 2+

PICK AND CHOOSE YOUR FAVORITE OPTIONS:

- Crackers
- French, sourdough, ciabatta, or Italian bread, sliced
- Olives
- Pickles
- Hummus
- Nuts
- Veggies (cucumbers, carrots, cherry tomatoes)
- Vegan deli meat rolled with ~1 TBSP vegan cream cheese
- Dried or fresh fruit

A winning charcuterie board experience is more about the presentation than fancy ingredients. Arrange your chosen nibbles on a large plate, cutting board, or pretty dish towel, and graze while studying or binge watching your favorite show.

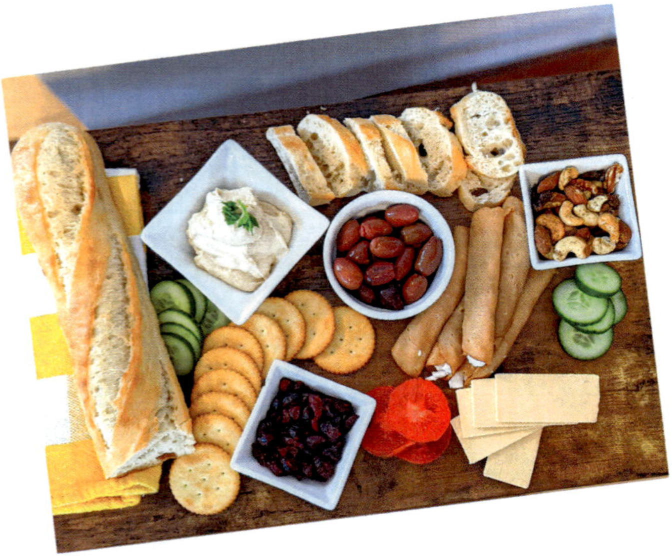

Did you know...?

Charcuterie is French for "fancy pork butcher" and describes a branch of cooking involving prepared meat products. We say it's high time to vegan-ize this 15th century tradition!

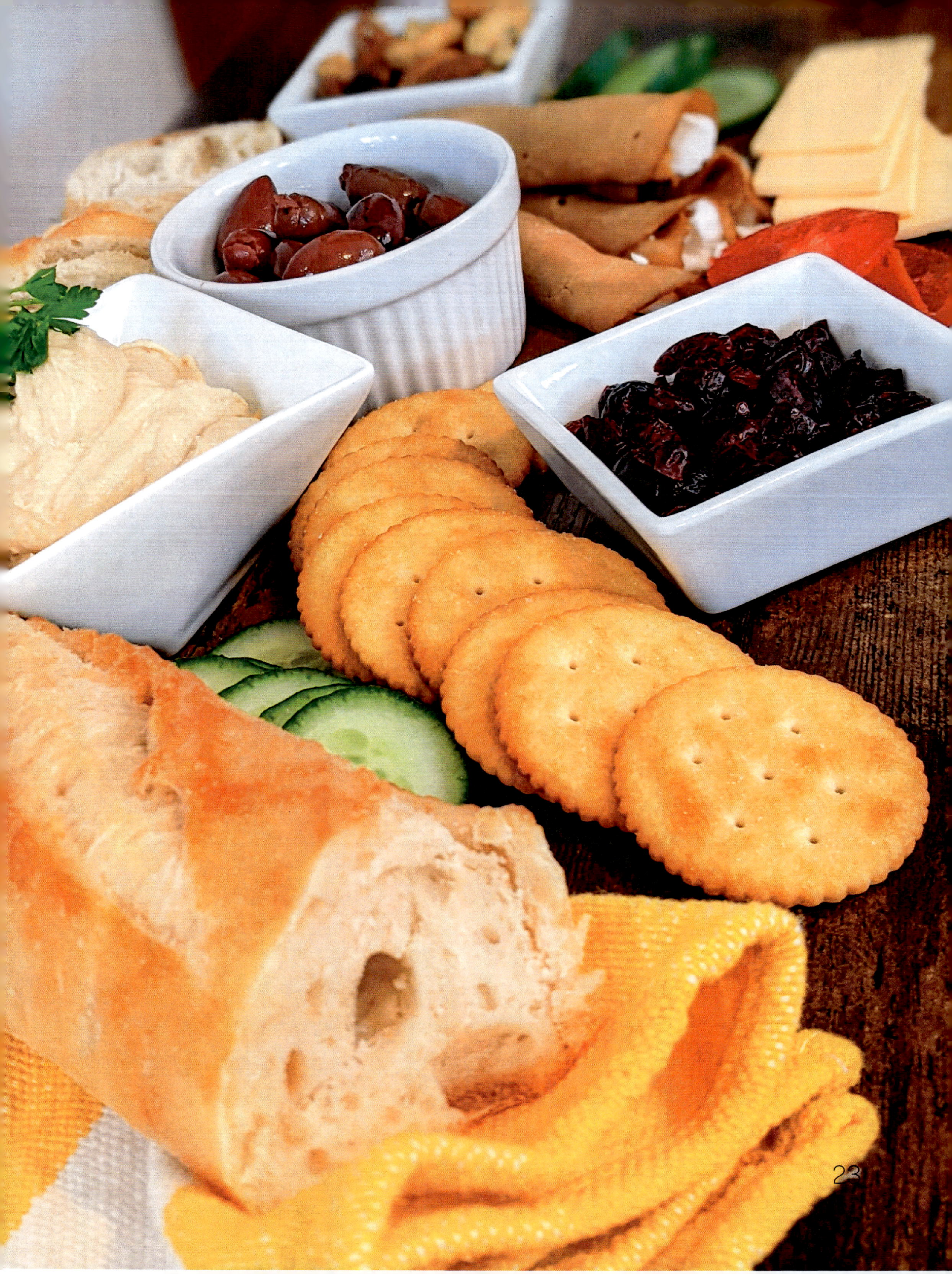

Cheater Guacamole

serves 1-2

- 1 ripe avocado (see notes)
- 1 TBSP chopped red onion
- Salt to taste

OPTIONAL:

- Cilantro, chopped
- Fresh lime juice
- 1 TBSP jalapeno, chopped

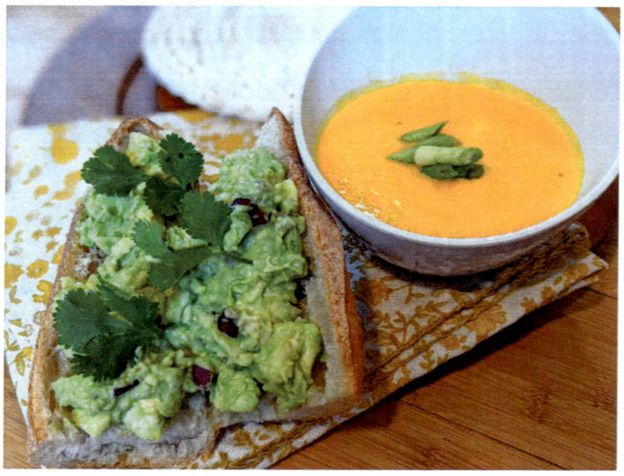

Slice open avocado and remove pit. Scoop the avocado flesh into a small bowl and add chopped red onion. Mash with a fork to desired consistency (we like ours chunky) and sprinkle with salt. Give it a taste and add more salt as needed.

Eat as is, with chips or veggies, on top of toast, or in a burrito (like our Hash Brown Burrito [page 40])!

NOTES: New to picking out avocados? Look for ones that are darker in color and have a slight give to them when you hold them in your hand. If you see any dents or the skin seems to pull away from the inside flesh, keep on moving - that one's too far gone!

Want to speed up the ripening process? Place inside a brown paper bag and leave on a counter or your desk for 1 to 2 days. Ripe before you need it? Pop it in the fridge!

This recipe is best when eaten right away. If you prepare ahead or have leftovers, place a piece of plastic wrap or foil directly over the guacamole to prevent air getting in and store in the fridge for up to 24 hours. (Adding a squeeze of lime juice will also help prevent browning.) Stir before eating.

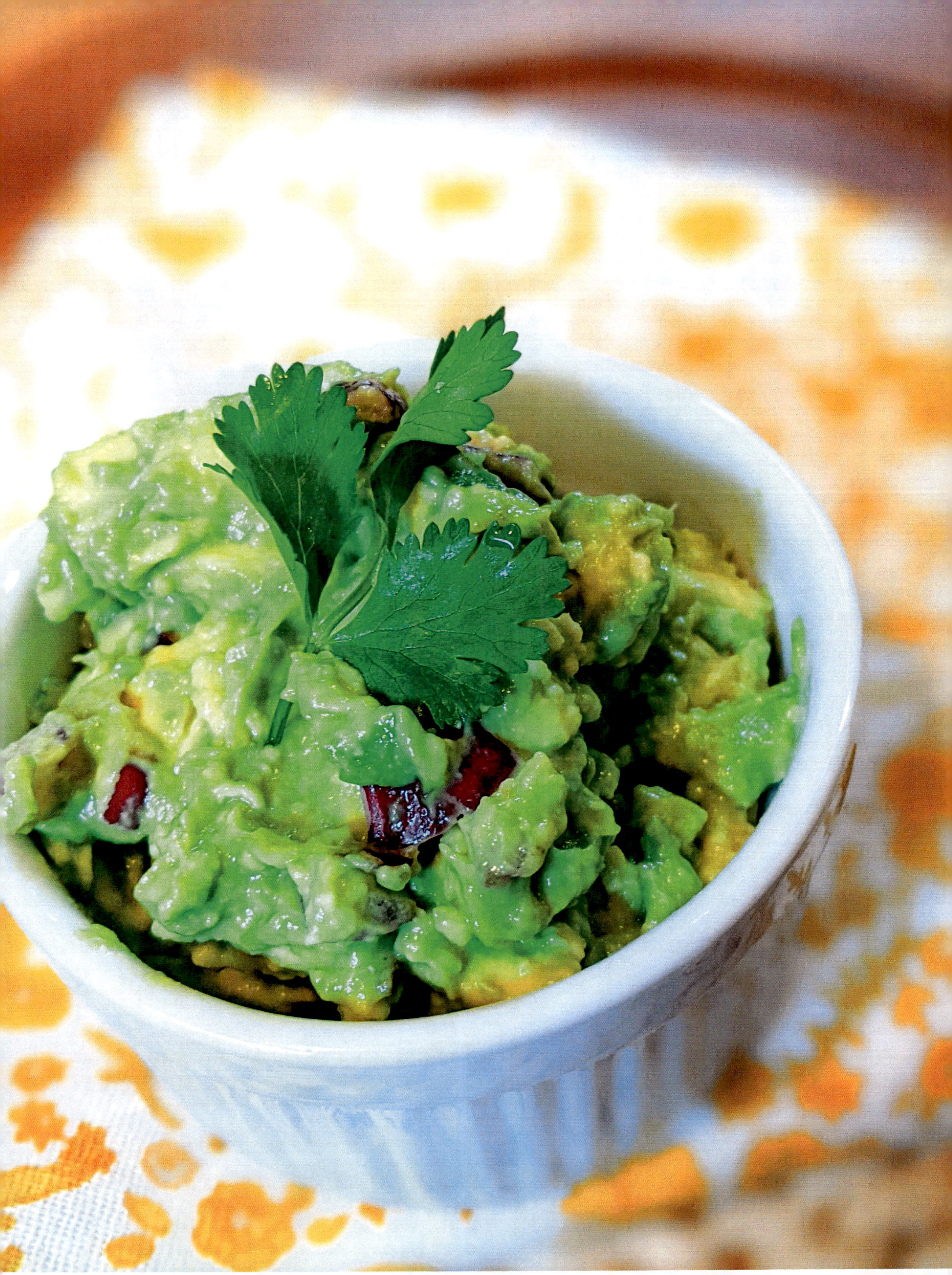

Easy Cheesy Dip

serves 2-4

- 1/2 package (about 4 oz) vegan cream cheese
- 1/2 cup (4 oz) salsa
- 1/4 cup scallions, sliced
- Tortilla or corn chips (for dunking)

In a microwave safe dish, combine cream cheese and salsa. Microwave on high for about 15-25 seconds, or until you can easily stir mixture until well blended. Add scallions and stir to incorporate. Dig in!

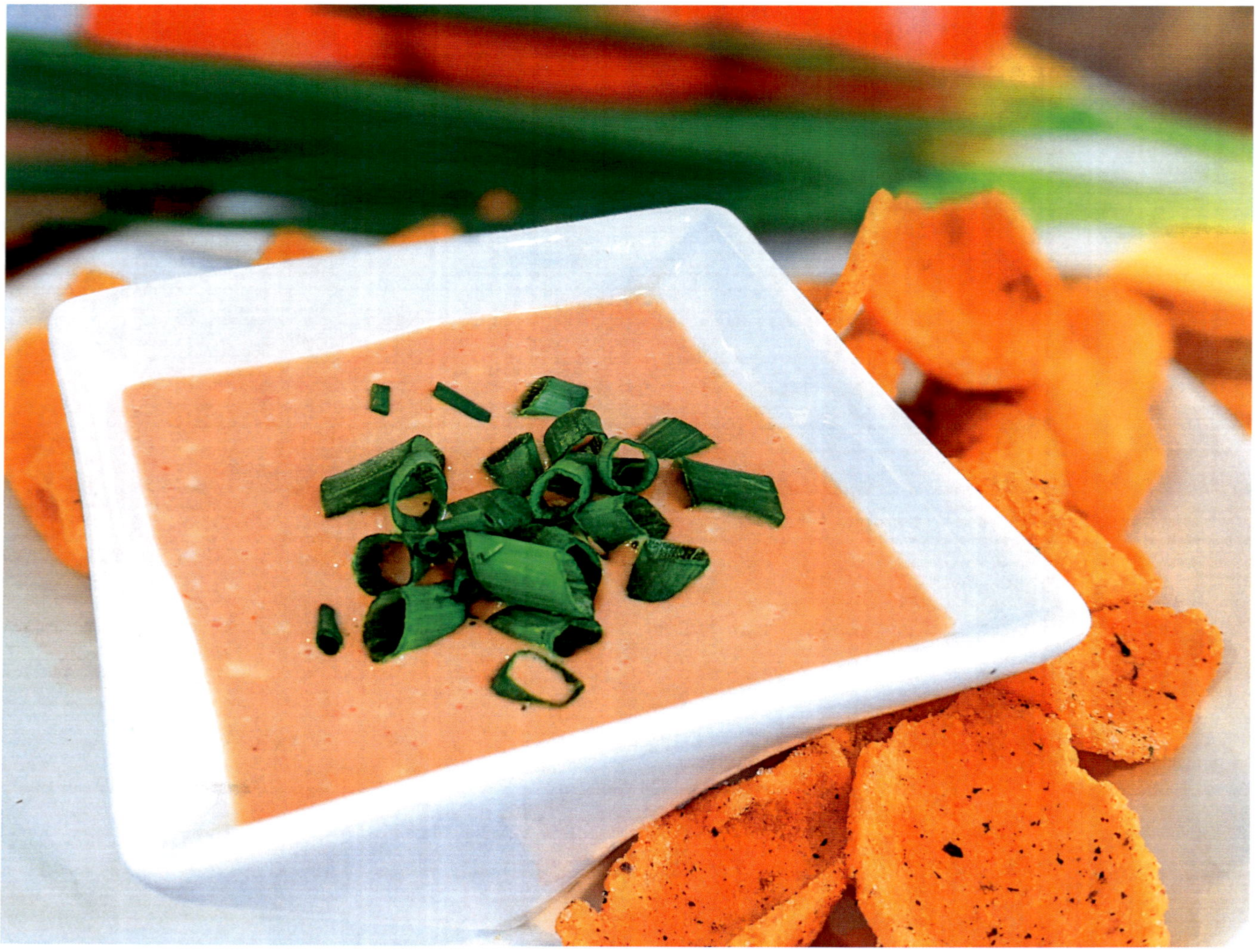

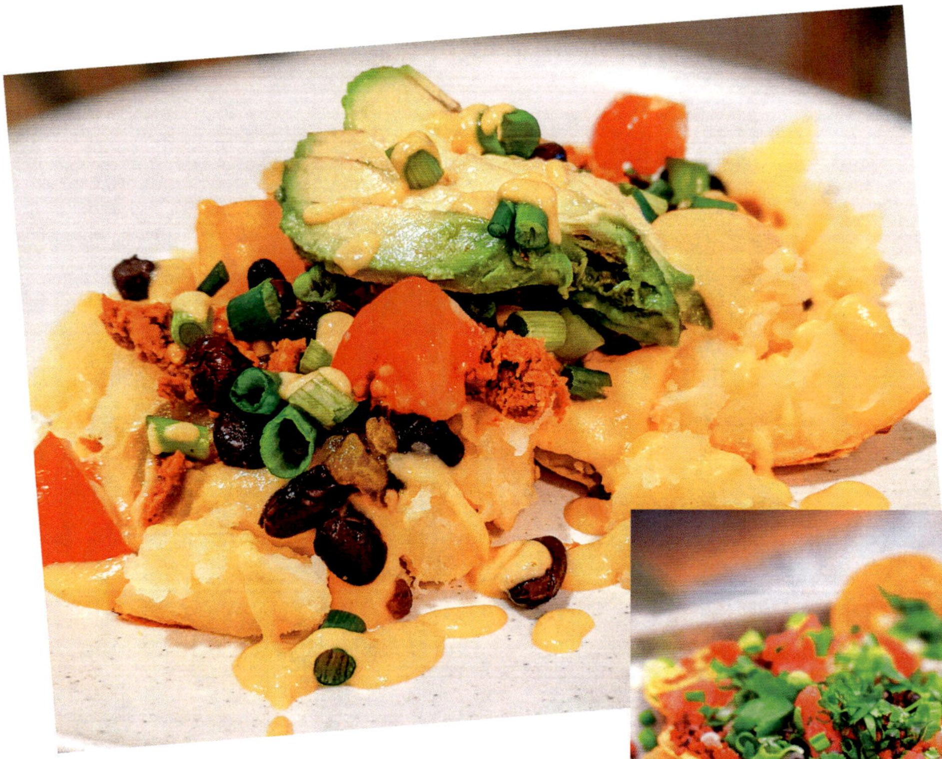

I'm versatile!

Try using this Easy Cheesy Dip in a baked potato bowl, nacho platter, burrito, quesadilla, or as a chopped salad dressing!

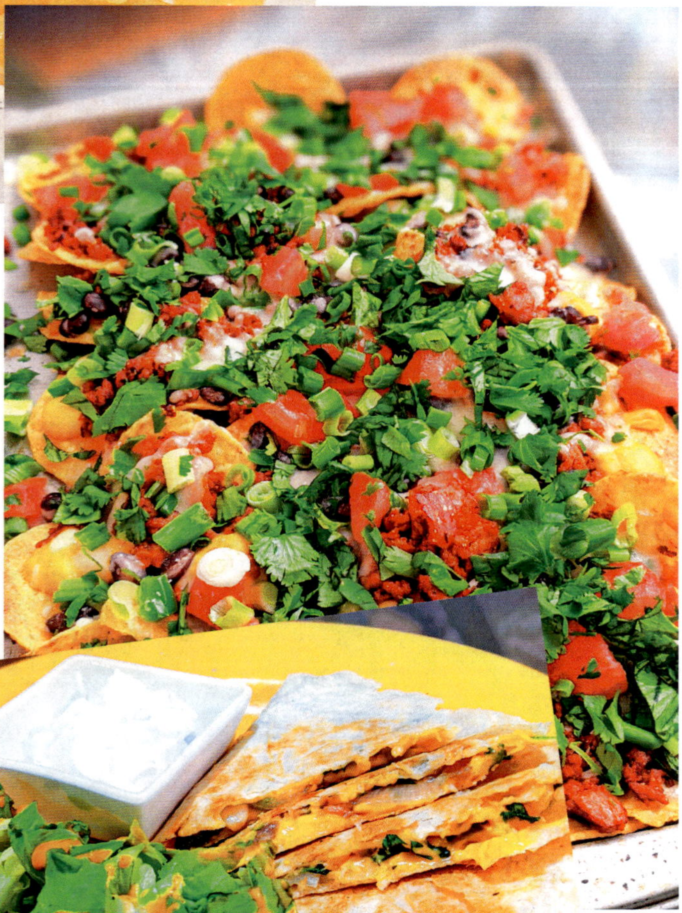

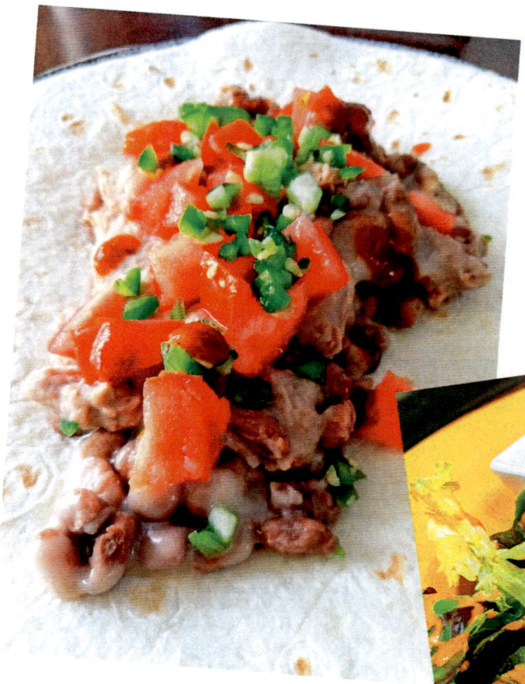

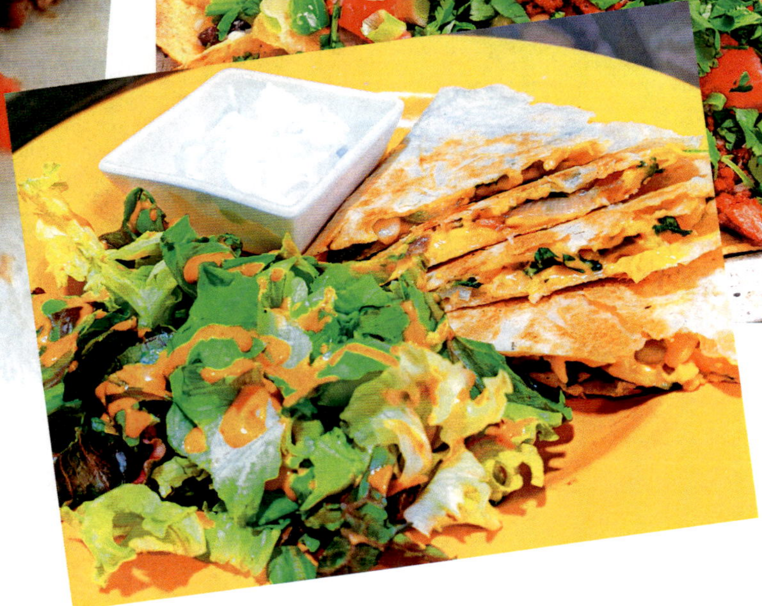

Fully Loaded Popcorn

serves 2+

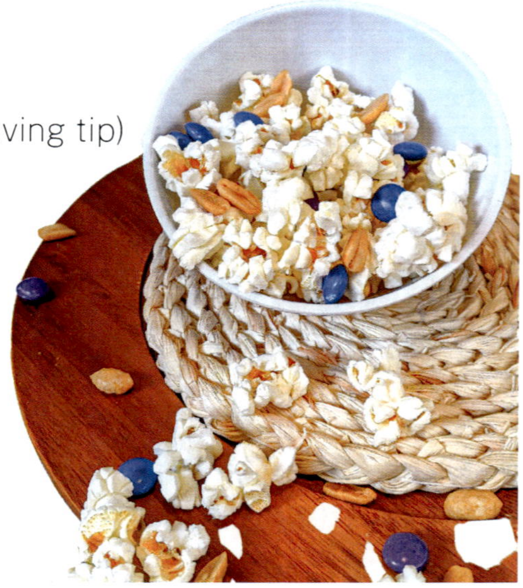

- 1 package microwave popcorn, popped (see money-saving tip)
- A large handful of vegan candy-coated chocolates
- A large handful of peanuts

OPTIONAL: Kettle Corn Glaze:

- 4 TBSP vegan butter
- 2 TBSP maple syrup or agave
- Sprinkle of cinnamon (optional)

If making glaze: In a microwave safe dish, combine vegan butter and maple syrup/agave. Microwave on high for about 30 seconds, or until butter is melted. Stir, and pour over your piping hot popcorn. You can add peanuts and chocolate candy before or after you pour glaze on. (If popcorn is in the microwave bag, give it a good shake after you pour on glaze.) Sprinkle cinnamon on top (if using) and dive in!

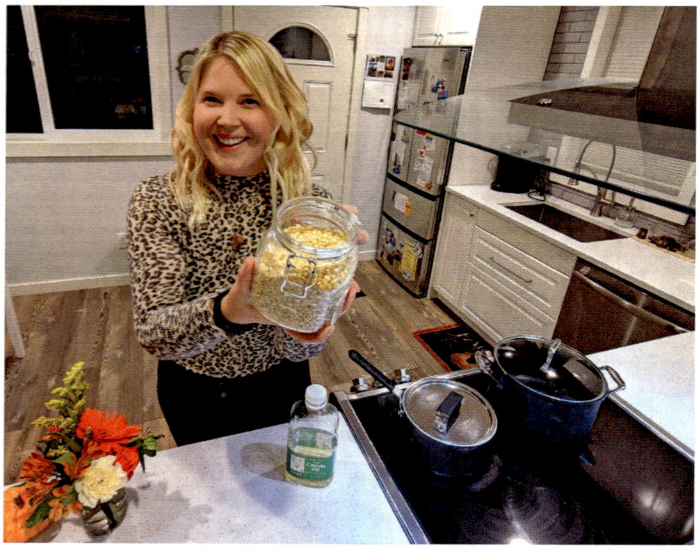

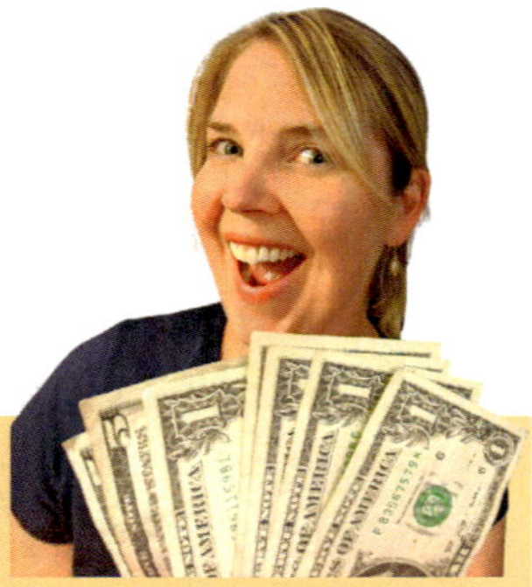

Money Saving Tip

If you purchase popcorn kernels in bulk and pop them on the stovetop, you can enjoy oodles of popcorn for pennies per serving! Visit our YouTube channel to watch how to do it in our Popcorn Hack Video!

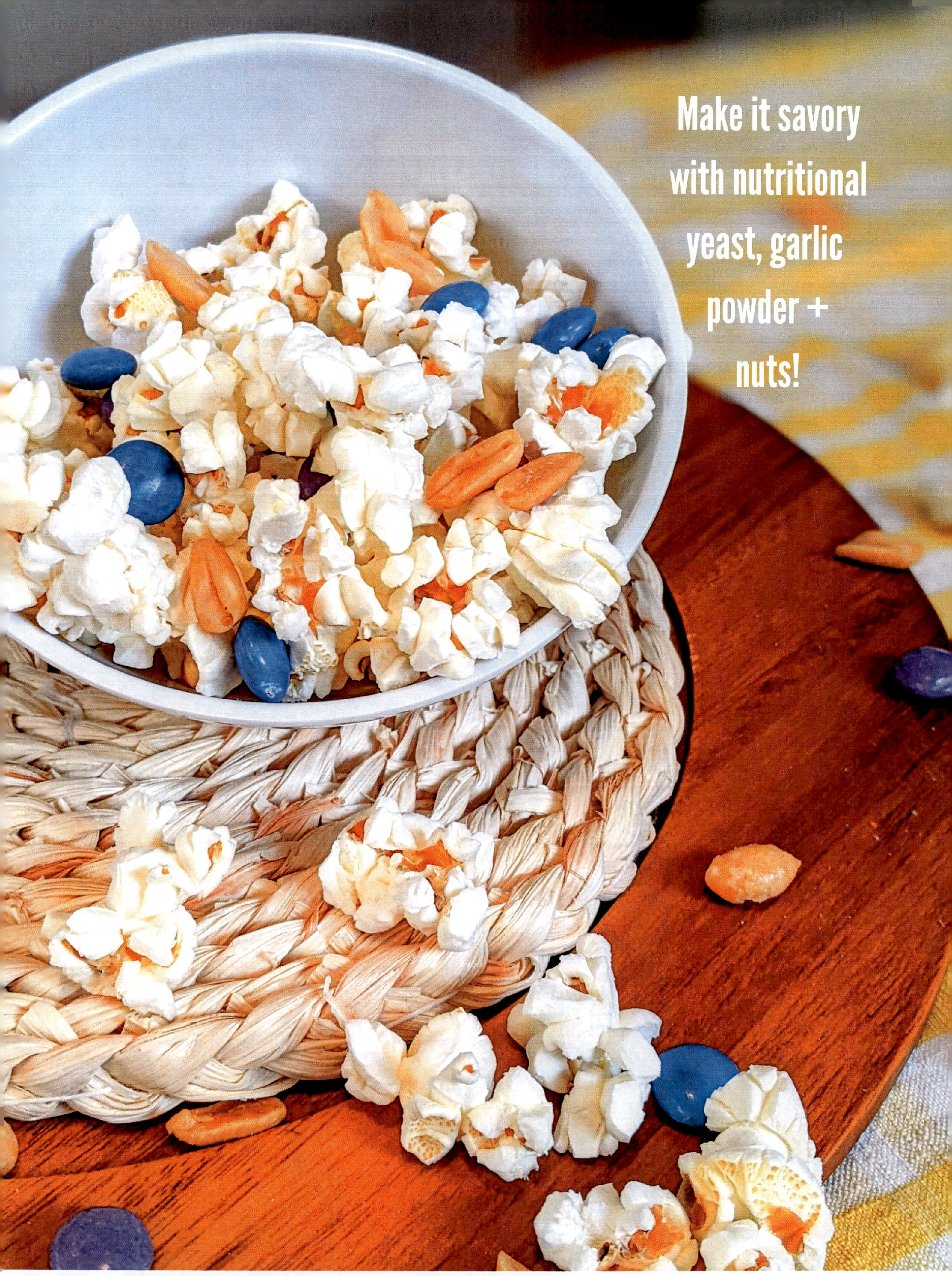
Make it savory
with nutritional
yeast, garlic
powder +
nuts!

Salad Dressing Hacks

serves 1-2 each

Base:

- 3-4 TBSP vegan mayo
- Dash of cracked pepper (optional)

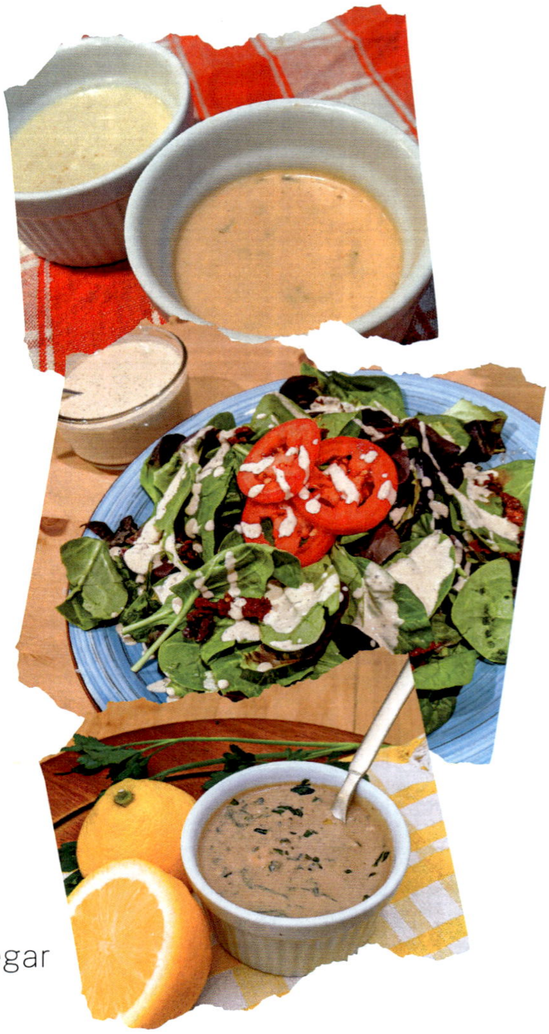

For "Honey" Mustard, add:

- 1 TBSP your favorite mustard
- 1 TBSP agave

For Thousand Island add:

- 1 TBSP relish
- 1 TBSP ketchup

For Ranch (see notes), add:

- 1 teaspoon dried dill
- 1/2 TBSP garlic powder

For Creamy Italian (see notes), add:

- 1 teaspoon red wine, white wine, or balsamic vinegar
- 1 teaspoon garlic powder
- 1 teaspoon dried basil
- 1 teaspoon dried oregano

Combine your chosen ingredients in a small bowl and give it a good stir. Use on salads, as a dipping sauce, or sandwich spread.

NOTE: Ranch and Creamy Italian dressings will taste best after being refrigerated for at least 4 hours (overnight is preferred). If you want to go the extra mile for the Ranch, consider adding dried parsley and chives, and/or a squeeze of fresh lemon juice.

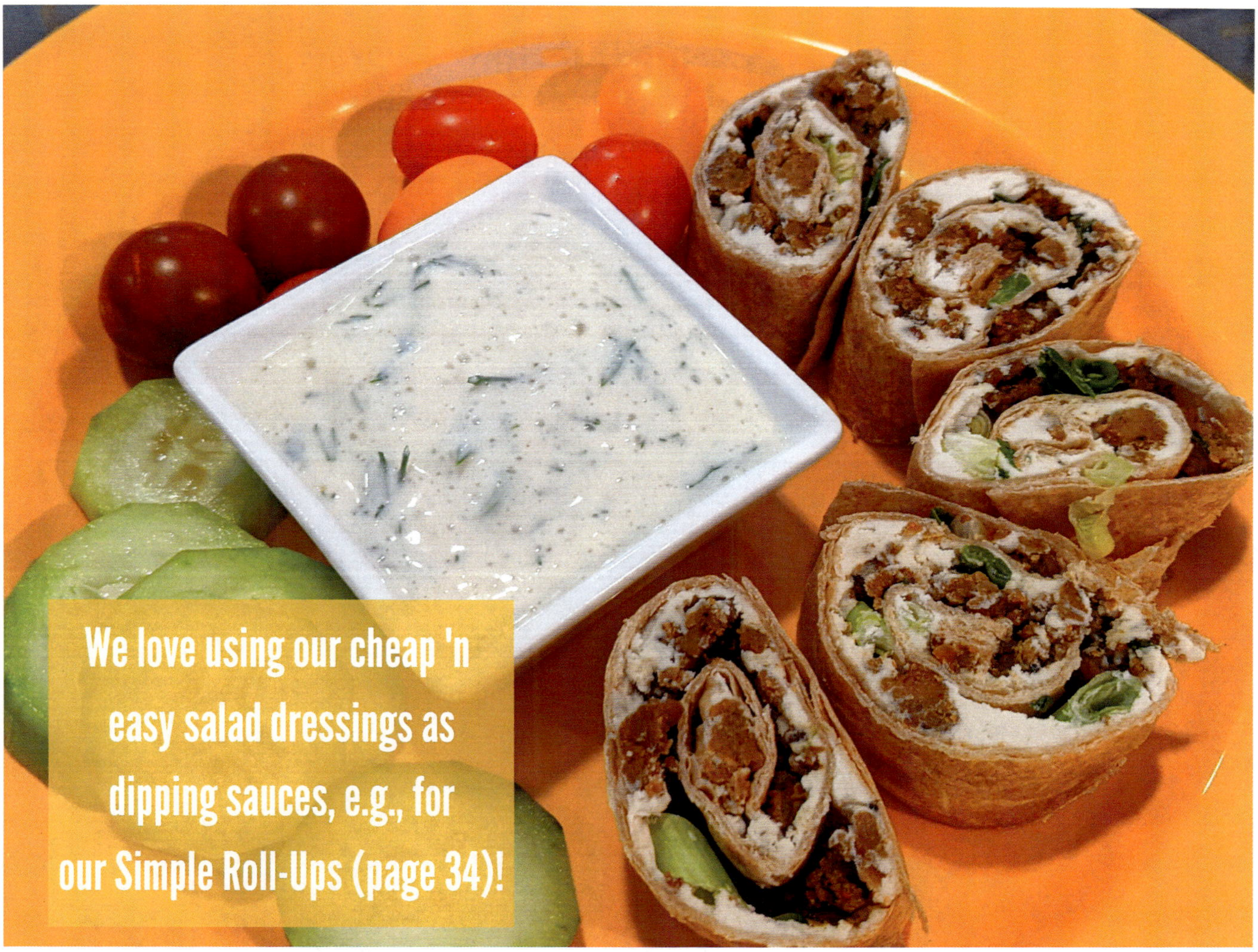

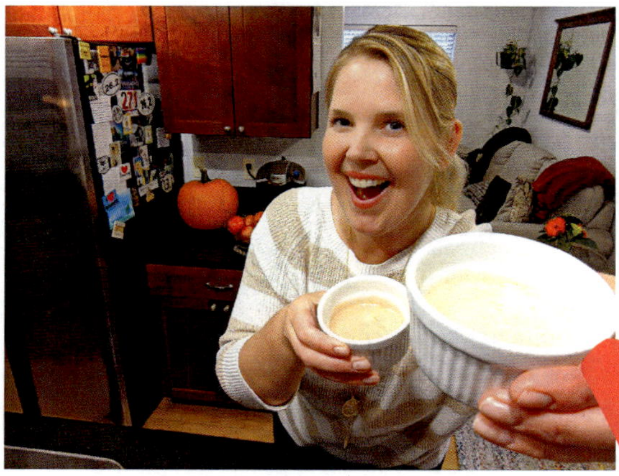

Watch the Video

If you're a visual learner, check out our YouTube channel and watch our "Dressing Up" video!

Simple Roll-Ups

serves 1

- 1 burrito-sized tortilla
- 4 TBSP vegan cream cheese
- 1-2 TBSP bell pepper (any color), finely chopped
- 1 TBSP scallions, sliced
- 1/4 cup vegan meat crumbles and/or vegan shredded cheese (optional)
- Salsa for dipping (optional)

Spread cream cheese in an even layer onto tortilla. Sprinkle all of your fillings inside in an even layer. Roll tightly into a tube, slice into bite-sized pieces, and enjoy!

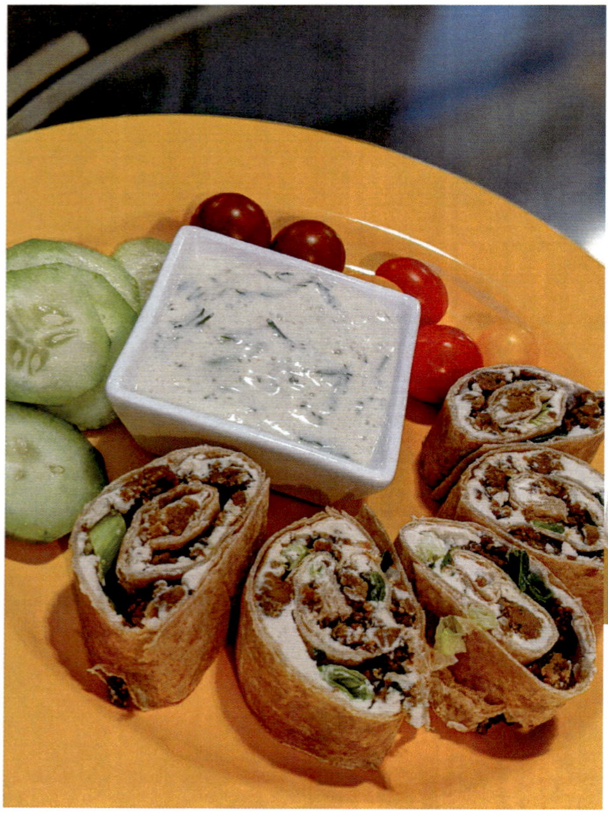

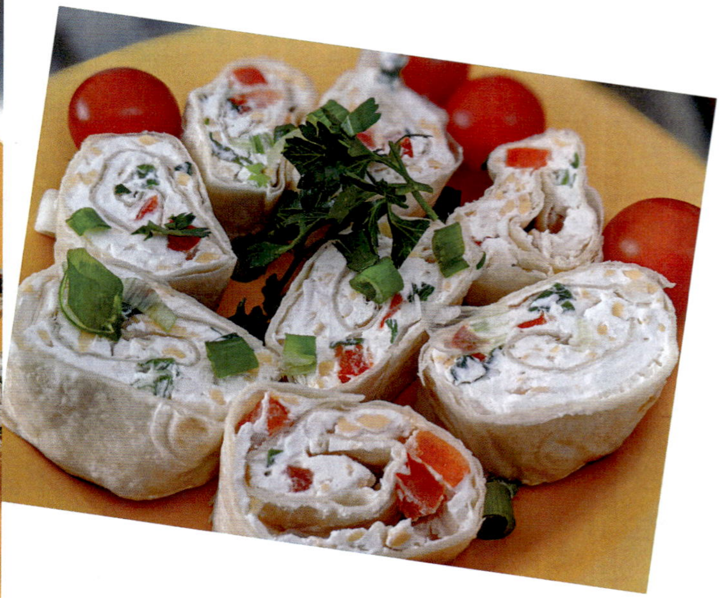

NOTES: You can also add vegan sour cream to your filling and play around with flavors; this is a great snack to share and keeps well in the fridge, so consider making extra!

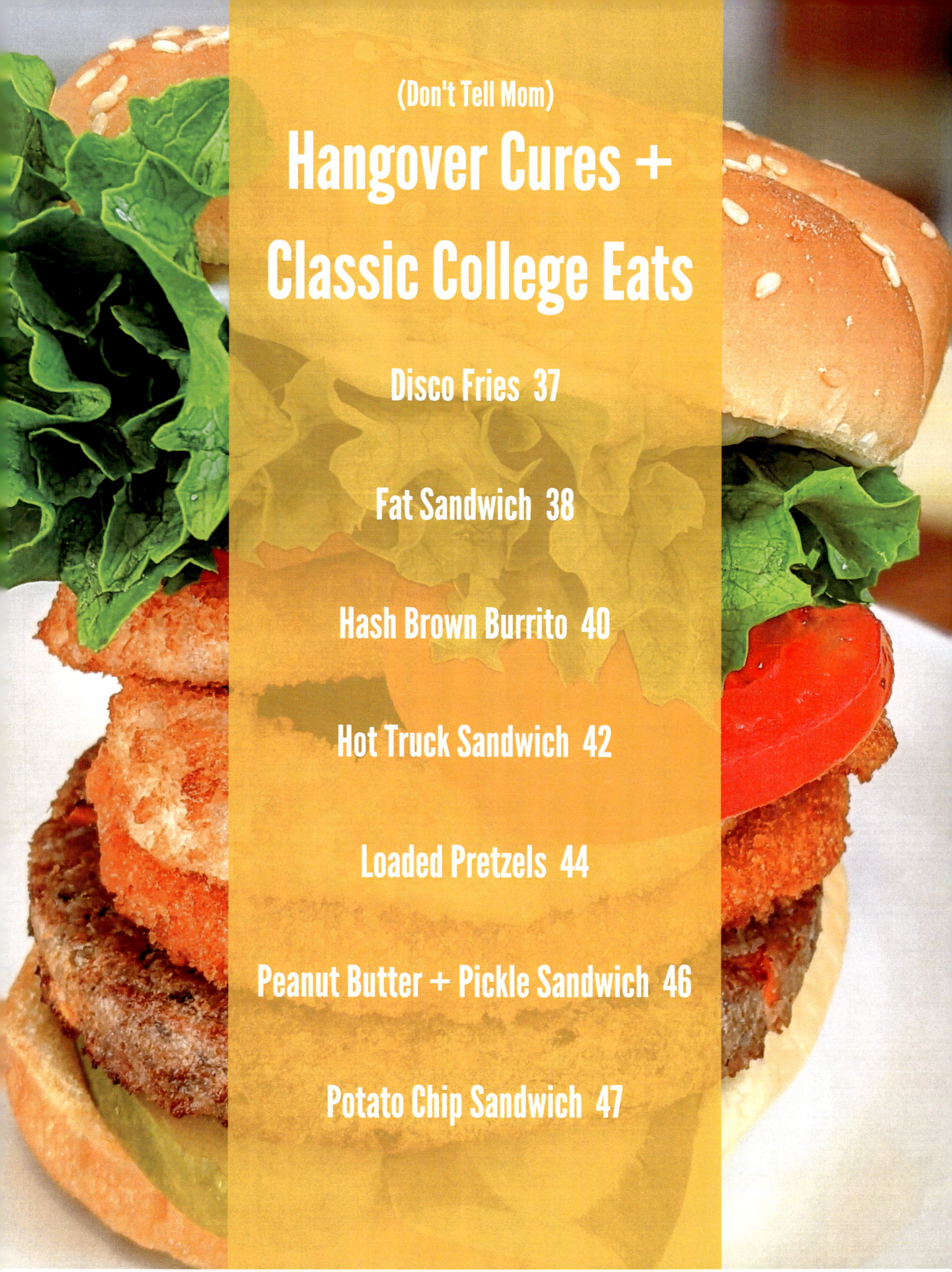

(Don't Tell Mom)

Hangover Cures + Classic College Eats

Psst...we interrupt this broadcast to bring you a note from...

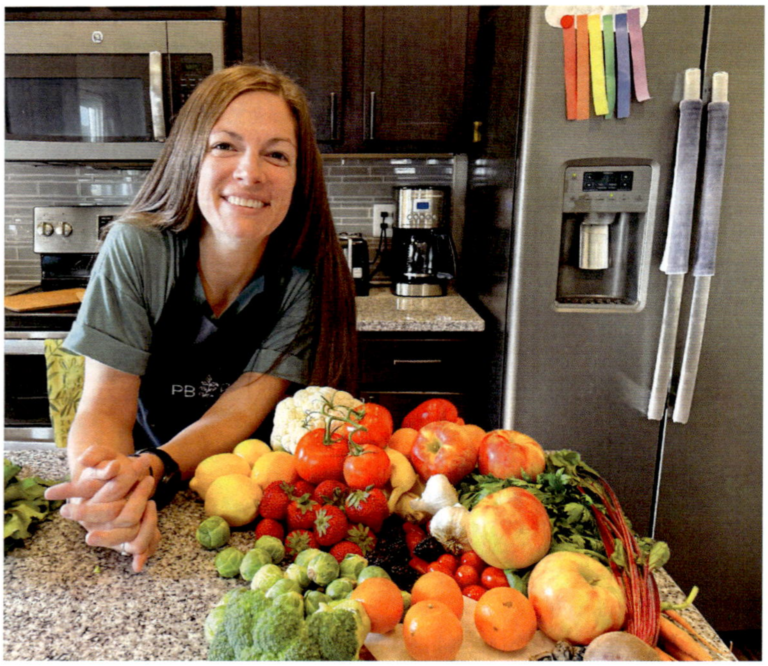

...Robin, our resident nutrition expert!

While all of the recipes in this section are sure to soak up some of that excess alcohol, we also want to give you some science-based guidance to help cure that hangover:

Hydration + Rest. Doesn't sound as fancy as a potato chip sandwich, BUT, the truth is: a lot of things are just band-aids and what our body really needs is some downtime + water.

Do your best to drink a glass of water before going to bed after an evening of cocktails and drink another glass as soon as you wake up.

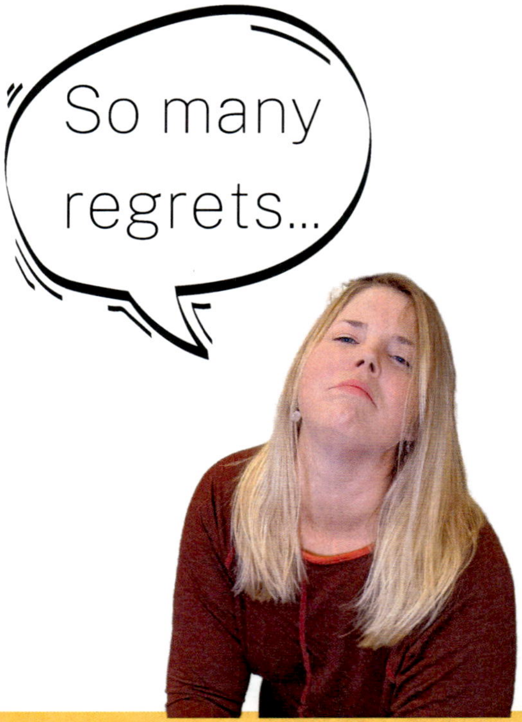

If your day allows, take a nap. These are not the days for a hard workout or cardio class.

And for snacks, think WATER-based foods:

- salads
- cucumbers
- oranges
- watermelon, etc.

Cheers!

Disco Fries

serves 1-2

- 1/2 package (13-oz) of your favorite frozen fries (or tots)
- 1/2 cup vegan gravy (see notes)
- 1/2 package vegan mozzarella cheese shreds

If you have access to a toaster oven or oven, cook fries according to package instructions, otherwise, you can microwave them until hot (though they won't be crispy). Heat gravy in microwave safe dish for 30-60 seconds (until warm). Place cooked fries on a microwave safe plate and pour warm gravy over top. Top with vegan mozzarella shreds, and microwave plate of disco fries until cheese is melted.

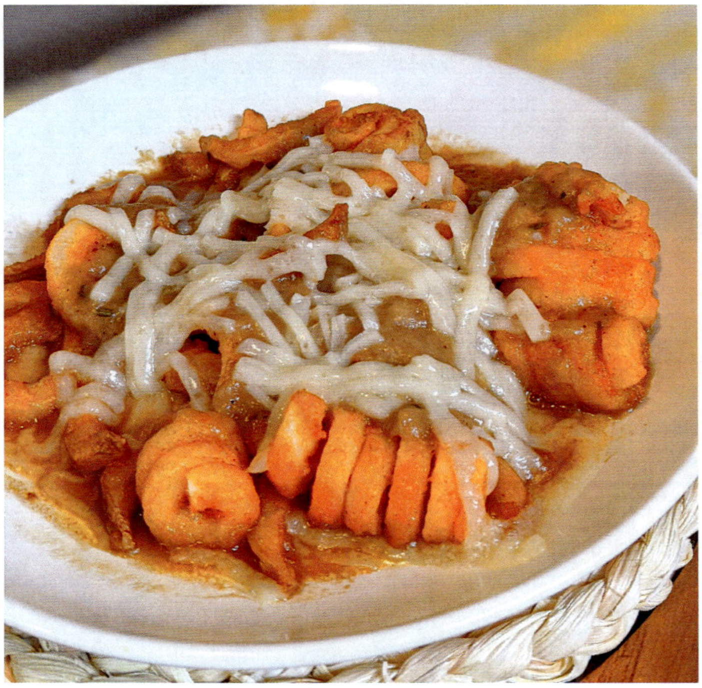

Did you know...?

This classic college eat originated in New Jersey and (in Jersey girl Jules's opinion) is far superior to poutine, the Canadian version which uses cheese curds instead of mozzarella.

NOTES: Many stores now sell packaged, ready-to-eat vegan/vegetarian gravy sauces. Jules likes to use the gravy packets that come with frozen vegan chick'n and turk'y products!

Fat Sandwich

serves 1

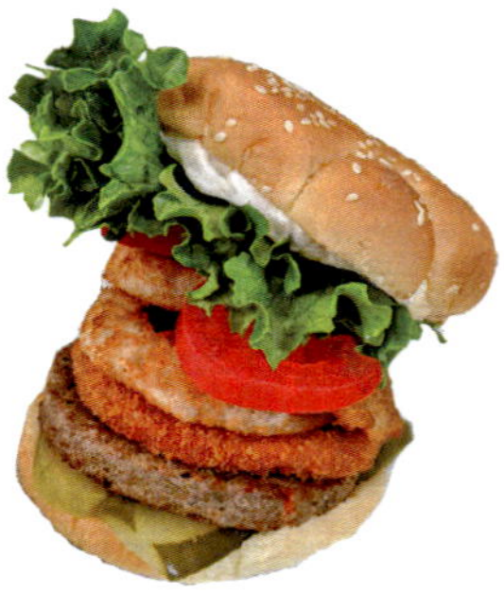

- 1 hamburger bun

CHOOSE YOUR FILLINGS:

- chick'n patty
- fishless patty
- meatless patty
- vegan cheese slice(s)
- onion rings
- french fries or tots

Jersey for the Win

This classic college eat originated on the Rutgers University campus in New Brunswick, NJ, and has been featured on numerous food shows.

CHOOSE YOUR CONDIMENTS:

- ketchup
- pickles
- mustard
- vegan mayo
- lettuce
- onion
- tomato
- avocado

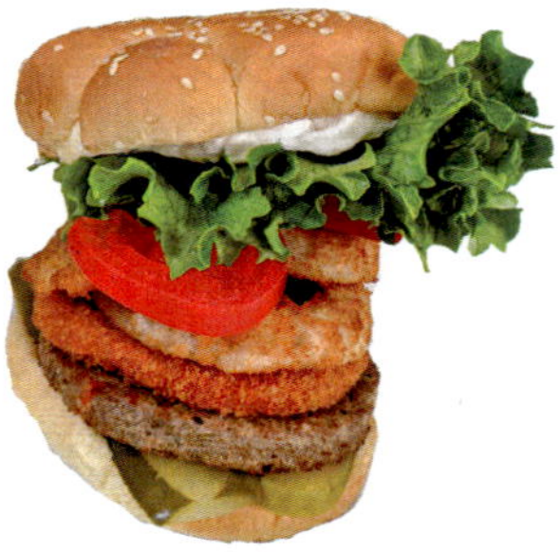

Microwave any of the vegan patties, onion rings, and/or fries you've chosen until heated through (optional: topped with vegan cheese). If you have access to an oven, toaster oven, or air fryer, feel free to use it to achieve a crisper outcome. Then layer together all of your chosen ingredients until your fat sammie is sky high.

And don't be limited by this list! The, er, sky's the limit.

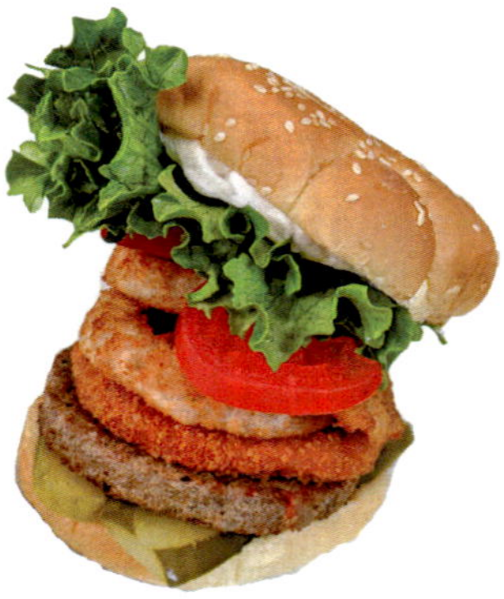

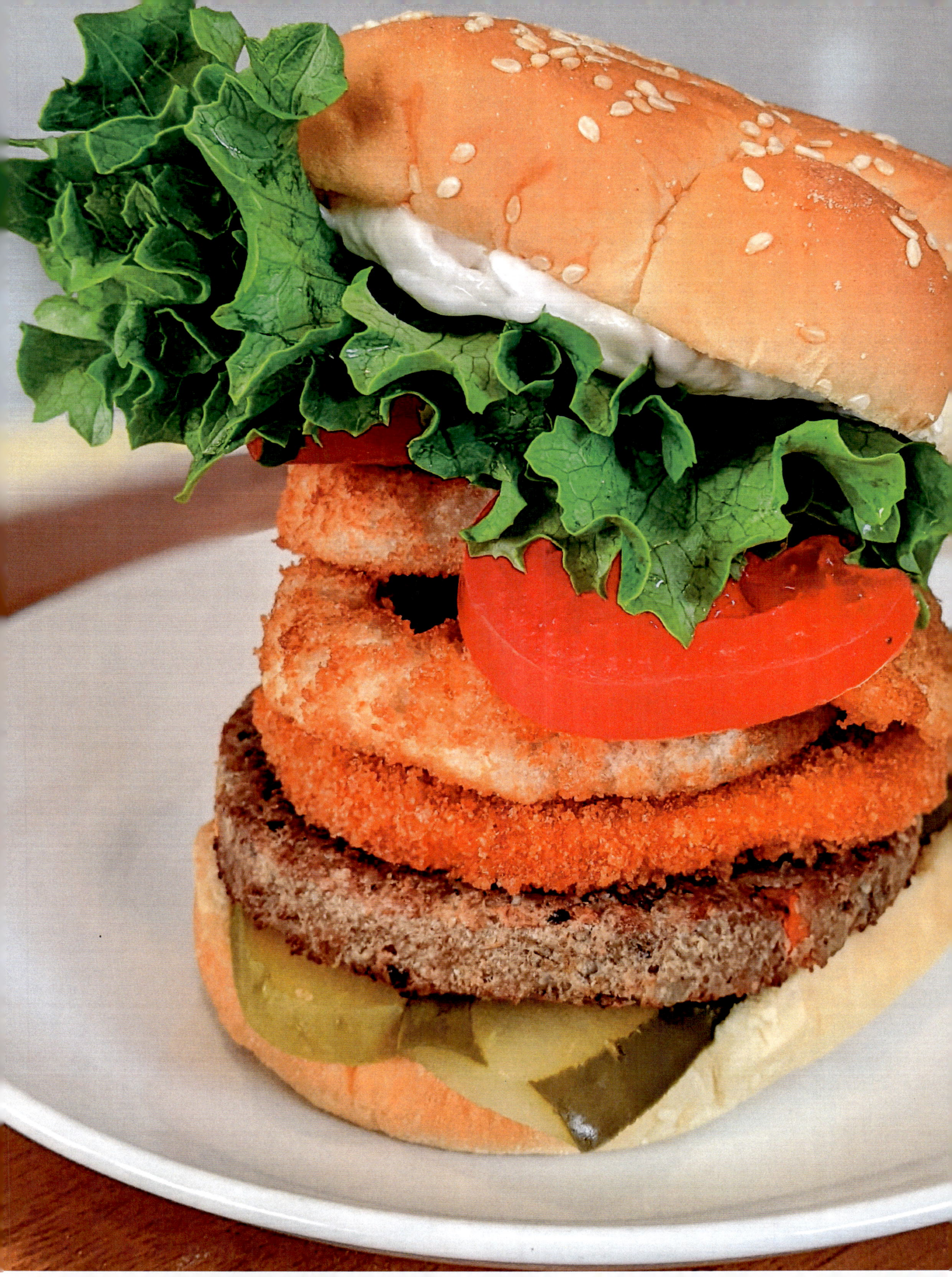

Hash Brown Burrito

serves 1

- 1 burrito-sized tortilla
- 3/4 cup hash browns or 1-2 hash brown patty (patties), cooked or warmed
- 1/2-1 avocado, mashed or sliced
- Sriracha, mustard, and or/ketchup to taste
- 1/2 cup black beans, rinsed (optional - see page 11 for our strainer hack)
- 1/4 cup vegan cheese shreds or slice of vegan cheese (optional)
- Salt and pepper to taste

Inside tortilla, pile all of your chosen ingredients and roll up using method pictured below. Microwave for an additional 30-60 seconds if desired.

Burrito Folding 101

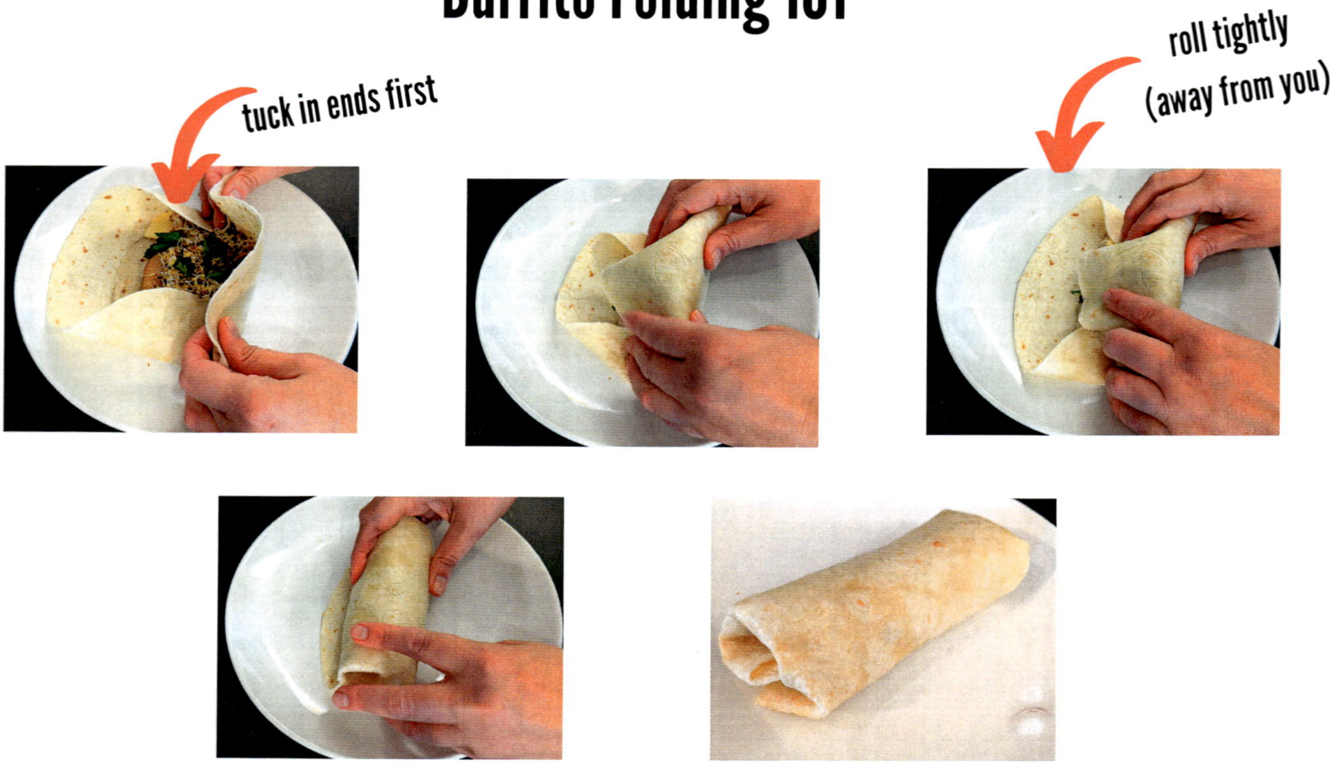

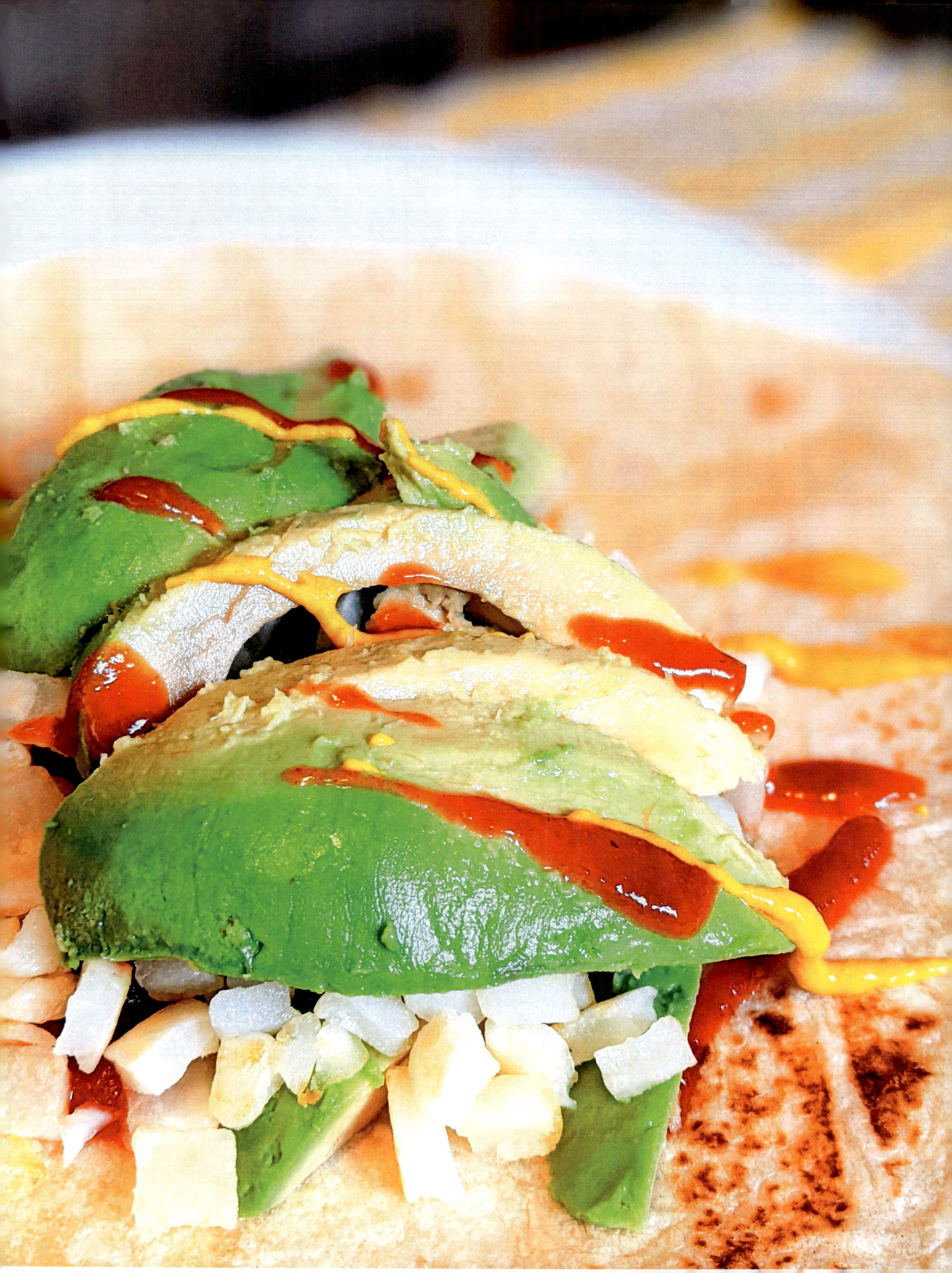

Hot Truck Sandwich

Needs Oven / Toaster Oven

serves 1-2

- One small loaf bread
- One small jar (8-15 ounces) pizza sauce
- 3/4-1 cup non-dairy mozzarella cheese
- 2 teaspoons fresh garlic -OR- garlic powder
- 2-4 TBSP vegan butter
- Toppings of your choice (spinach, tomatoes, etc.)

Preheat oven or toaster oven to 350 degrees Fahrenheit.

Cut bread in half and sprinkle garlic powder and melted vegan butter on each half. If using fresh garlic, chop and combine with melted vegan butter, then spread on bread.

Bake bread for 10 min on a baking sheet (vegan butter side up).

Once bread is done toasting, add to each side: tomato sauce, non-dairy mozzarella cheese, toppings of choice. Put the loaf back together (carefully) and wrap with aluminum foil (optional).

Return loaf to oven for four minutes. Let cool and enjoy!

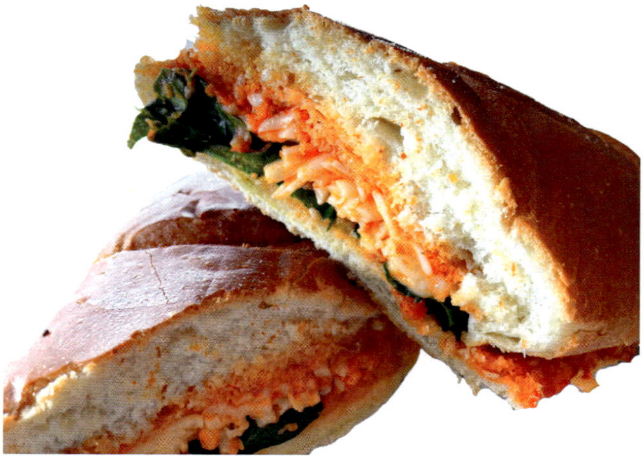

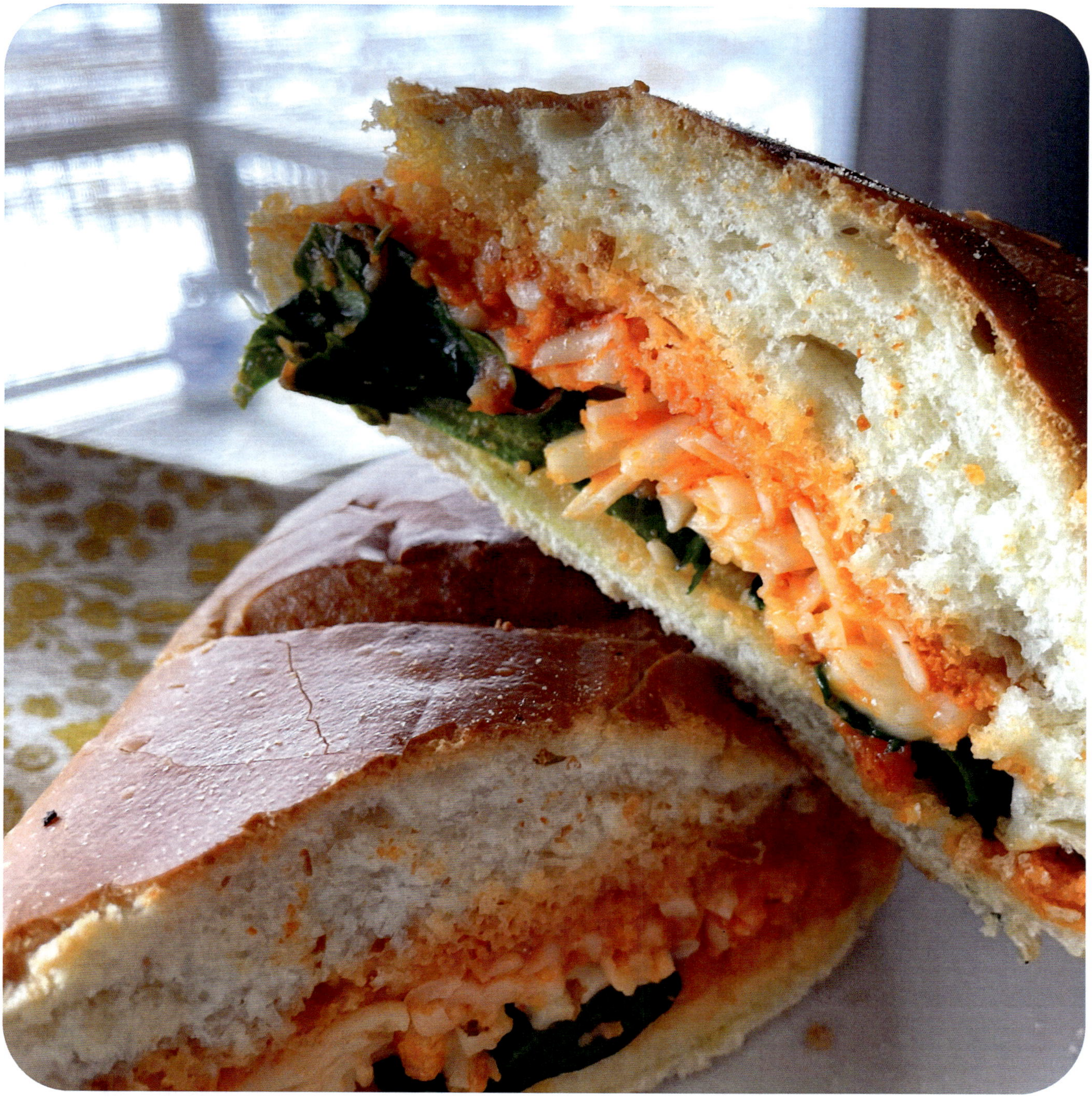

Who doesn't love pizza in a sandwich? A good friend shared this hot truck sandwich classic, and with some vegan magic, we found a perfect way to still enjoy this cheese-filled prize while checking the vegan box - voila! A go-to on cold nights with nothing but studying and statistics ahead of you.

Loaded Pretzels

serves 1-2

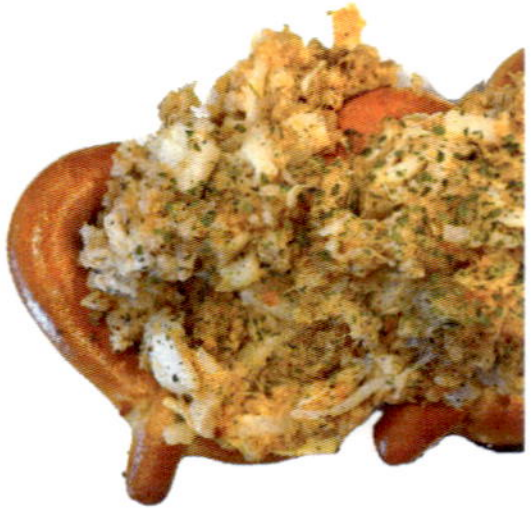

- 3-4 frozen pretzels, prepared according to package instructions
- Hearts of palm (1 14-oz can), drained and moisture squeezed out - can substitute artichokes or jackfruit
- 1/4-1/2 cup vegan mayo
- 1/4 cup bread crumbs, or more to taste (see notes)
- Salt and pepper to taste
- Old Bay seasoning to taste (see notes)
- Optional: add some nutritional yeast or non-dairy cheese shreds

In a bowl, mash hearts of palm with a fork. Add spices, bread crumbs, and vegan mayo and stir to combine. (Use more or less depending on whatever you like!) Pile on top of cooked pretzels and dig in!

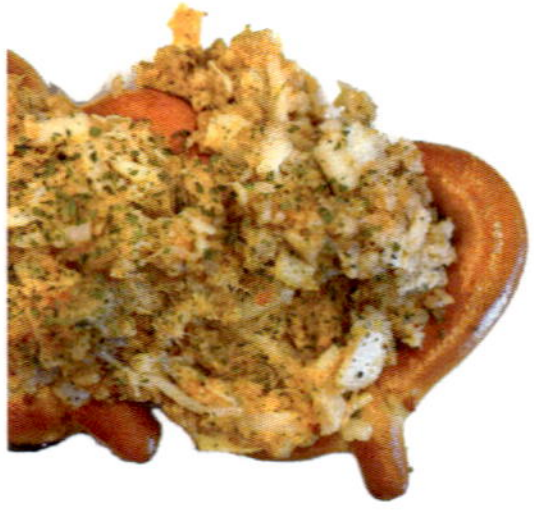

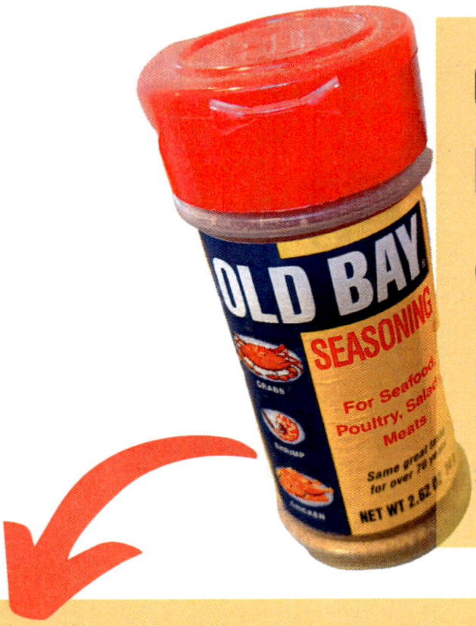

Old Bay, 'tis the seasoning of Maryland

Old Bay is a staple in most homes in Maryland (and beyond). Most notably for the unique spice blend that adds a seafood flavor to your seafoodless meals.

NOTES: To make your own Old Bay seasoning for this recipe, combine: ½ tsp celery salt (or ½ tsp celery seed + ¼ tsp salt), ½ tsp paprika, a pinch of crushed red pepper or cayenne pepper, and a few turns of black pepper.

Many store-bought breadcrumbs contain milk, so be sure to check the ingredients label. (Panko breadcrumbs are generally accidentally vegan.) It's also very easy to make your own breadcrumbs. To yield about 1/4 cup breadcrumbs, dry out or toast one slice of your favorite bread, and, if the bread is dry enough, you can crumble by hand!

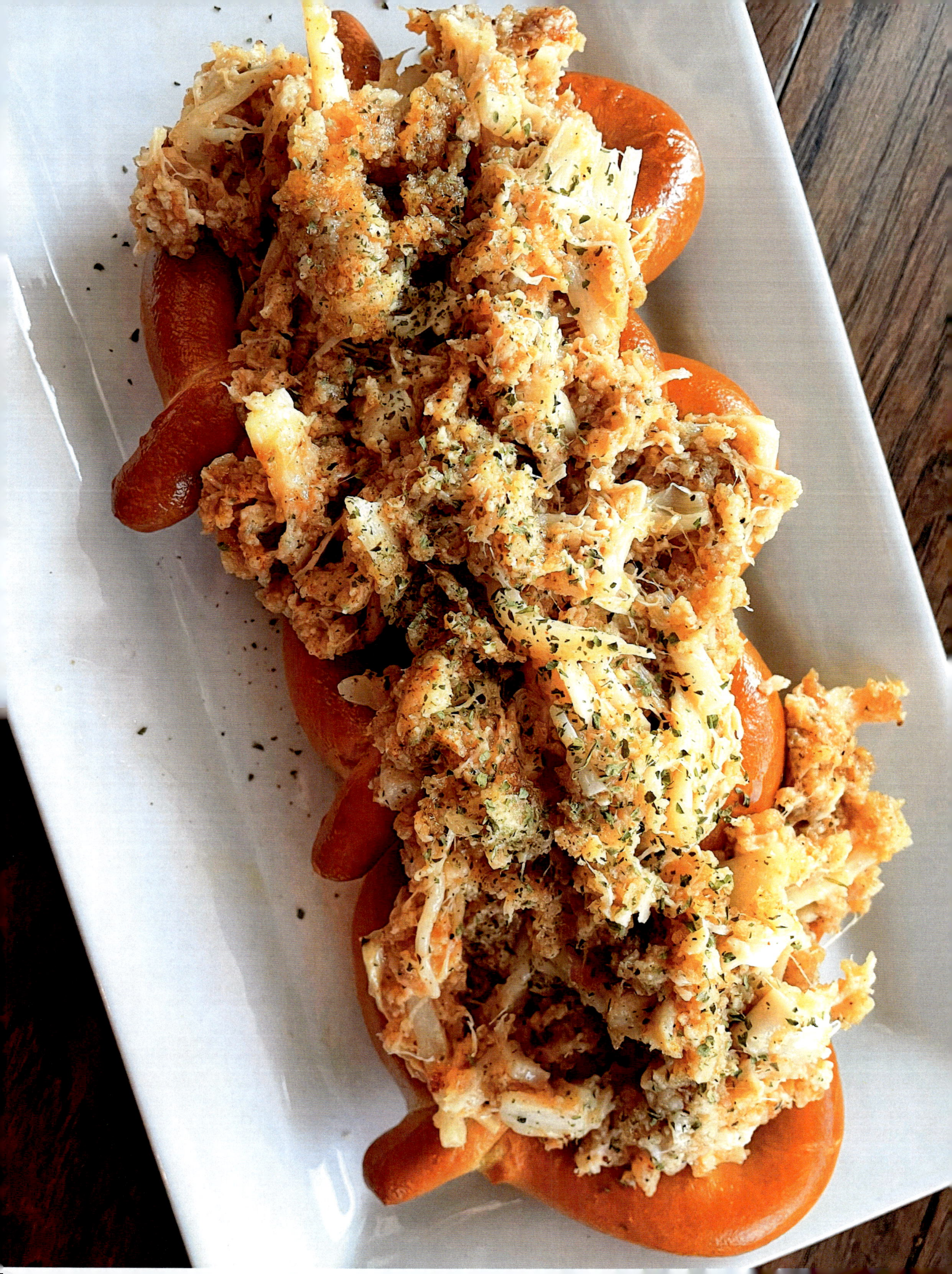

Peanut Butter + Pickle Sandwich

serves 1

- 2 slices of your favorite bread
- 4-6 TBSP of your favorite peanut butter
- 3-4 large pickle slices (sweet or dill)

Generously coat both slices of bread with peanut butter, and top one side with pickle slices. (We prefer dill!) Place two bread slices together, and slice on the diagonal if you're feeling fancy. Dig in!

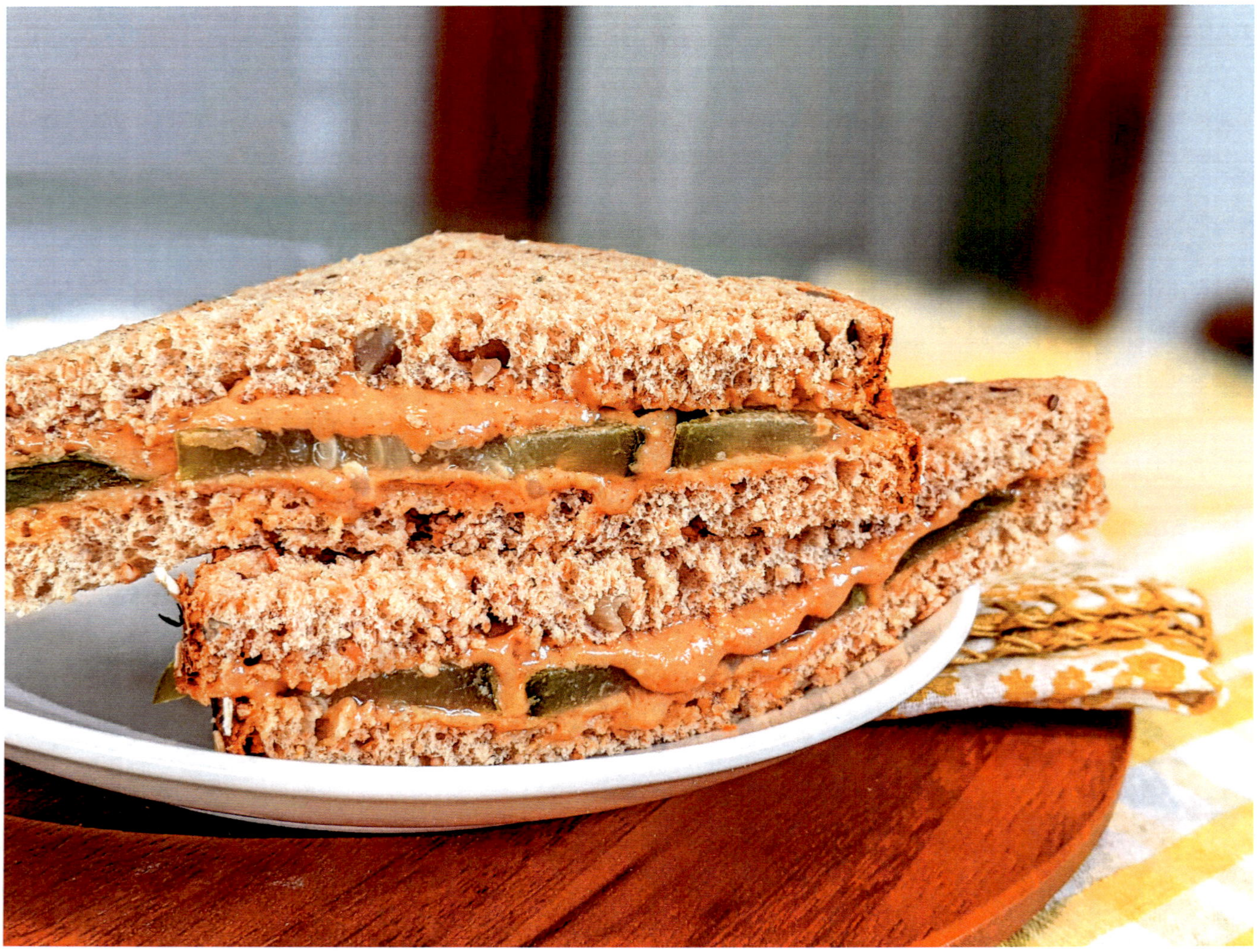

Potato Chip Sandwich

serves 1

- 1 hamburger roll (or 2 slices of your favorite bread)
- 2-3 TBSP vegan mayo or butter
- Large handful of potato chips

Generously coat roll or bread with vegan mayo or butter. (We prefer mayo!) Place a large handful of potato chips inside, and then give it a good SMOOSH.

Feeling crazy? Combine this with the Peanut Butter + Pickle Sandwich or Fat Sandiwch!

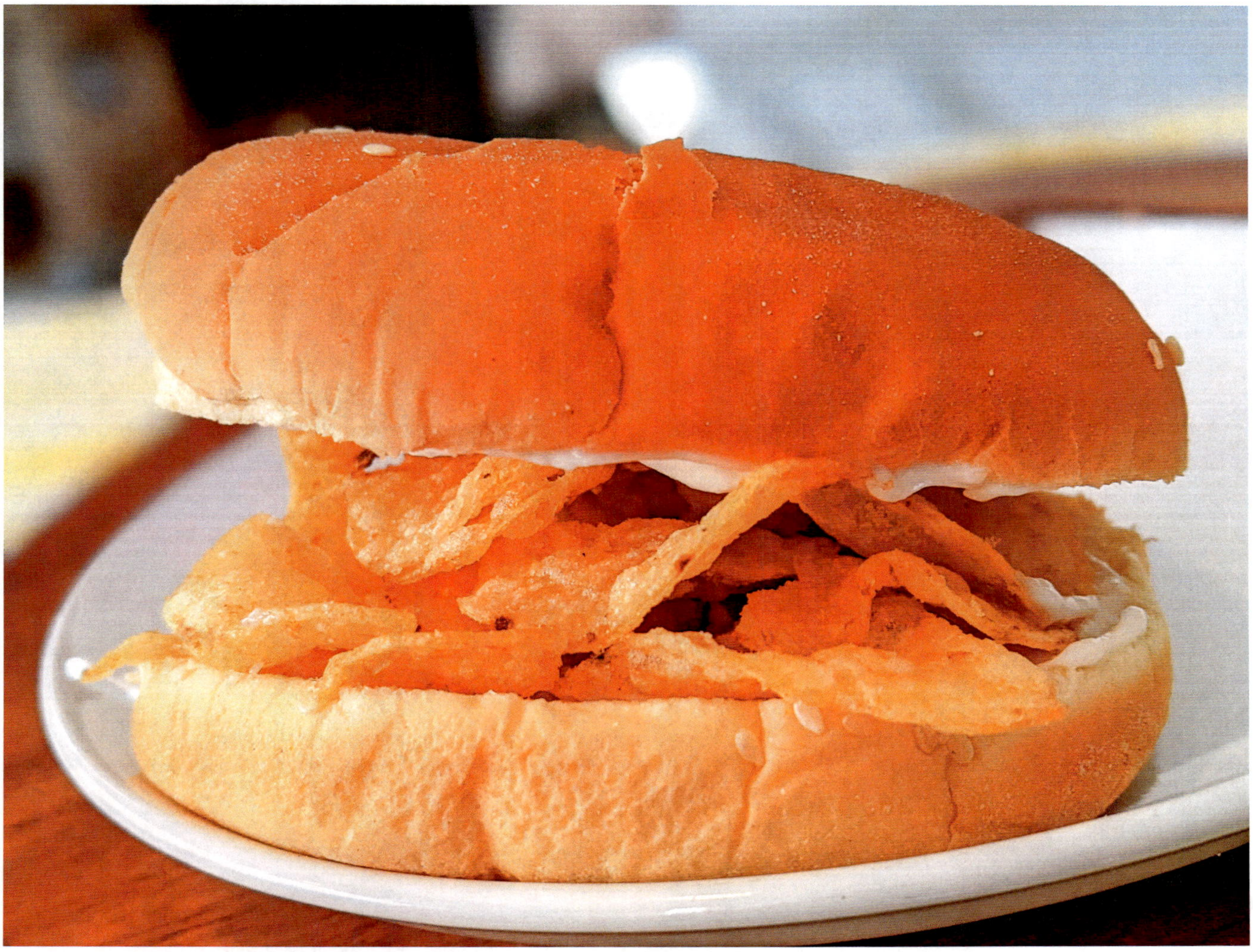

Meals

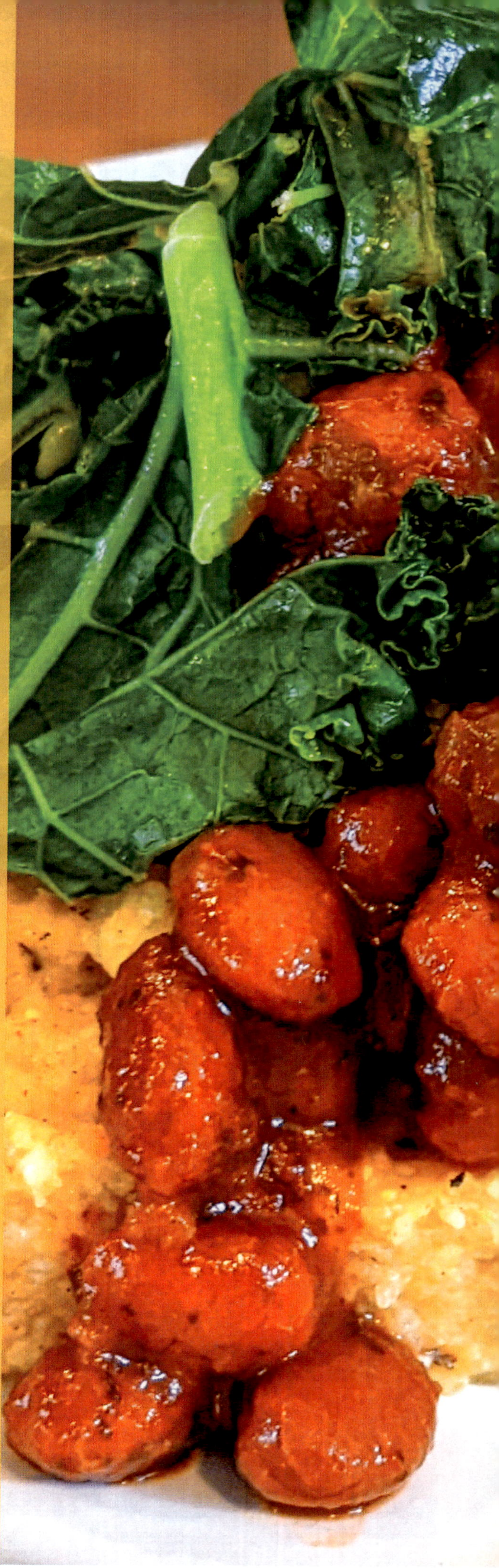

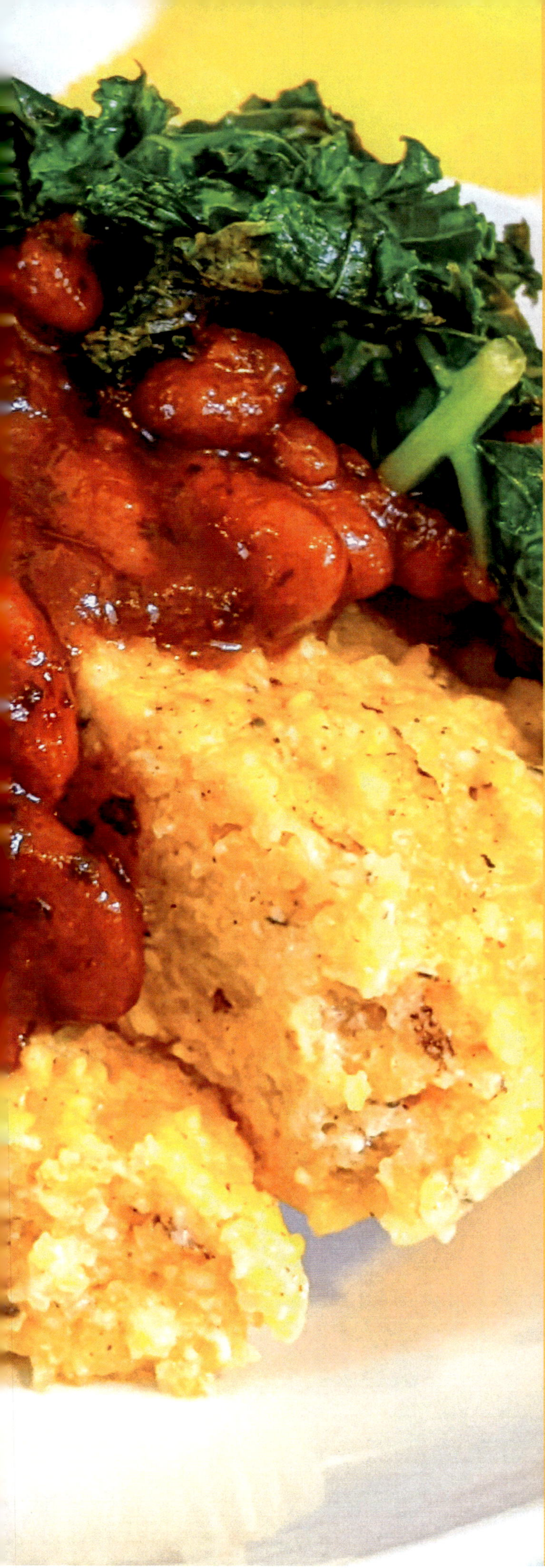

BBQ Chickpea Salad Boats

serves 2

- 1 15-oz can chickpeas, drained and rinsed (see page 11 for our strainer hack)
- 3-4 TBSP BBQ sauce
- 3-4 TBSP vegan mayo
- 1/2 cup frozen corn, thawed (can also use fresh or canned)
- 6-10 butter, romaine, or leafy lettuce slices ("boats"), rinsed and patted dry

OPTIONAL ADD-INS:

- 1/4 cup sliced scallions
- 10-12 cherry tomatoes, halved or quartered
- 2-3 TBSP chopped pickles or relish
- Salt and pepper to taste

In a medium-sized bowl, combine all ingredients except lettuce slices and stir until well mixed. Scoop a large spoonful into each lettuce slice/"boat" and dig in. If this is too messy, feel free to chop lettuce and make a salad! (Or pop it all into a burrito/wrap.)

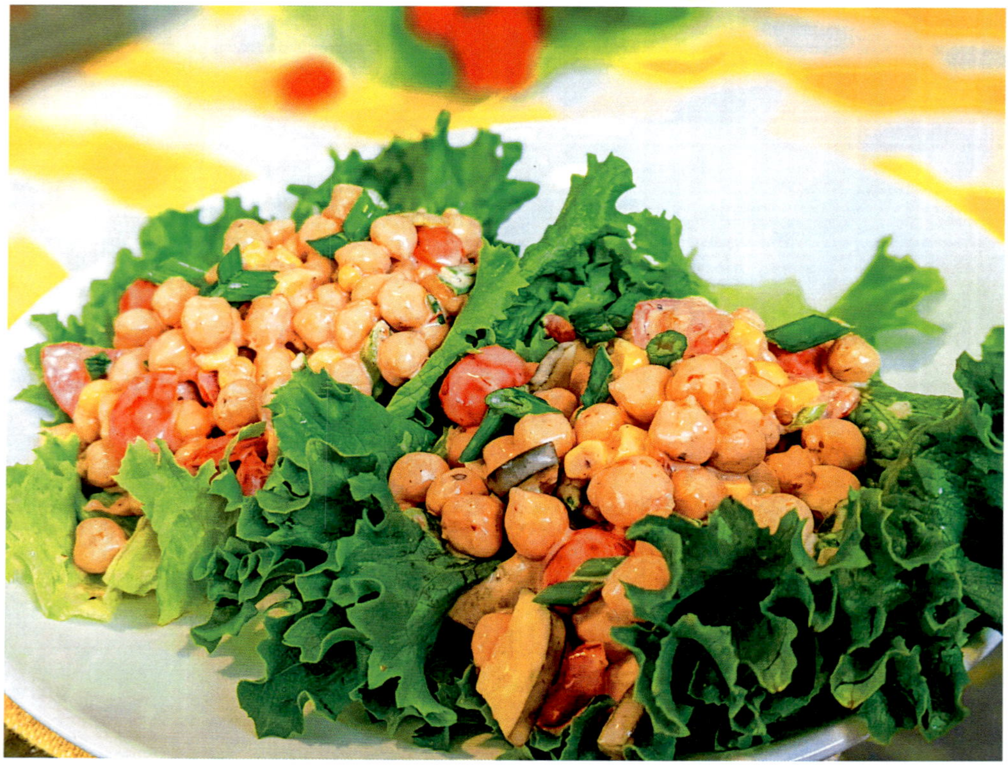

Bean Burritos

serves 2

- 2 burrito-sized tortillas
- 1 can vegan/vegetarian refried beans, heated

OPTIONAL ADD-INS:

- Hot sauce and/or salsa
- 1/4 cup chopped red onion, tomatoes, scallions, and/or jalapeno
- 1/2 cup vegan cheese shreds

Inside each tortilla, scoop half a can of your heated refried beans. Top with any optional toppings, roll-up (see page 40 for burrito rolling tips), and enjoy! If you have a stove/stovetop, you can also easily turn this into quesadillas (page 72) or enchiladas (page 52)!

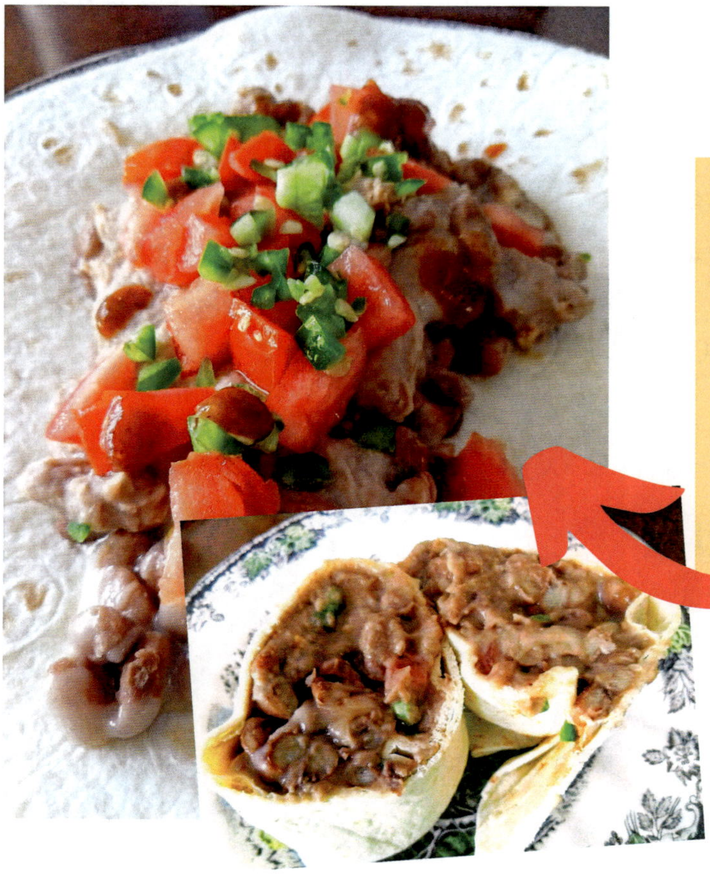

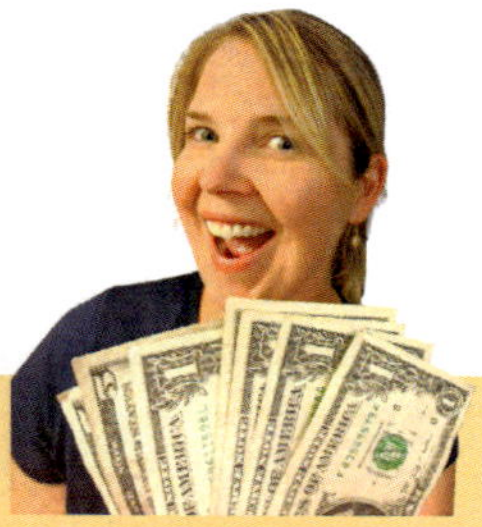

Money Saving Tip

If you have access to a pressure cooker and food processor, you can buy dried pinto beans and make your own DELICIOUS refried beans for pennies! Check out our YouTube channel and watch the Refried Beans Hack video!

Needs Oven

Cheater Enchiladas

serves 6

- 6 burrito-sized tortillas

FILLING (see notes):
- 1 can black, kidney, or pinto beans, rinsed and drained (see page 11 for our strainer hack)
- 2 cups rice, cooked
- 2 cups hash browns or cubed potatoes (white or sweet), cooked
- 1/2 cup sliced scallions (optional)
- 1/2 cup corn (optional)

This recipe is for the chefs out there; for a simpler option using similar ingredients, see our Bean Burrito (page 51) and Quick Quesadilla (page 72) recipes.

CHEATER ENCHILADA SAUCE:
- 1 15-oz can plain tomato sauce/tomato puree
- 1 TBSP each: garlic powder, onion powder + oregano
- Sprinkle of crushed red pepper or cayenne pepper (optional)

TOPPING (optional):
- 1 cup vegan shredded cheese or nutritional yeast

Preheat oven (or large toaster oven) to 375 degrees Fahrenheit (see notes). Prepare desired filling ingredients and set aside. In a small bowl, mix together enchilada sauce ingredients and set aside. Scoop 1/6th of the filling into each tortilla. (You can layer your filling ingredients as you go, or combine them in a large bowl first.)

Roll-up each burrito (see page 40 for burrito rolling tips), and place into a large 9x13-inch baking dish. Top with enchilada sauce (and vegan cheese/nutritional yeast if using). Bake for 30 minutes. Remove from oven and let cool for 5-10 minutes before digging in.

NOTES: Almost any filling you can dream up will work as an enchilada filling, and will impact the labor/cost. For example, we also love soy chorizo and vegan beef/chick'n, but those can get pricy.

If you want to try this in a microwave, you can halve the recipe and place 2-3 enchiladas into a large, microwave safe dish and microwave until heated through.

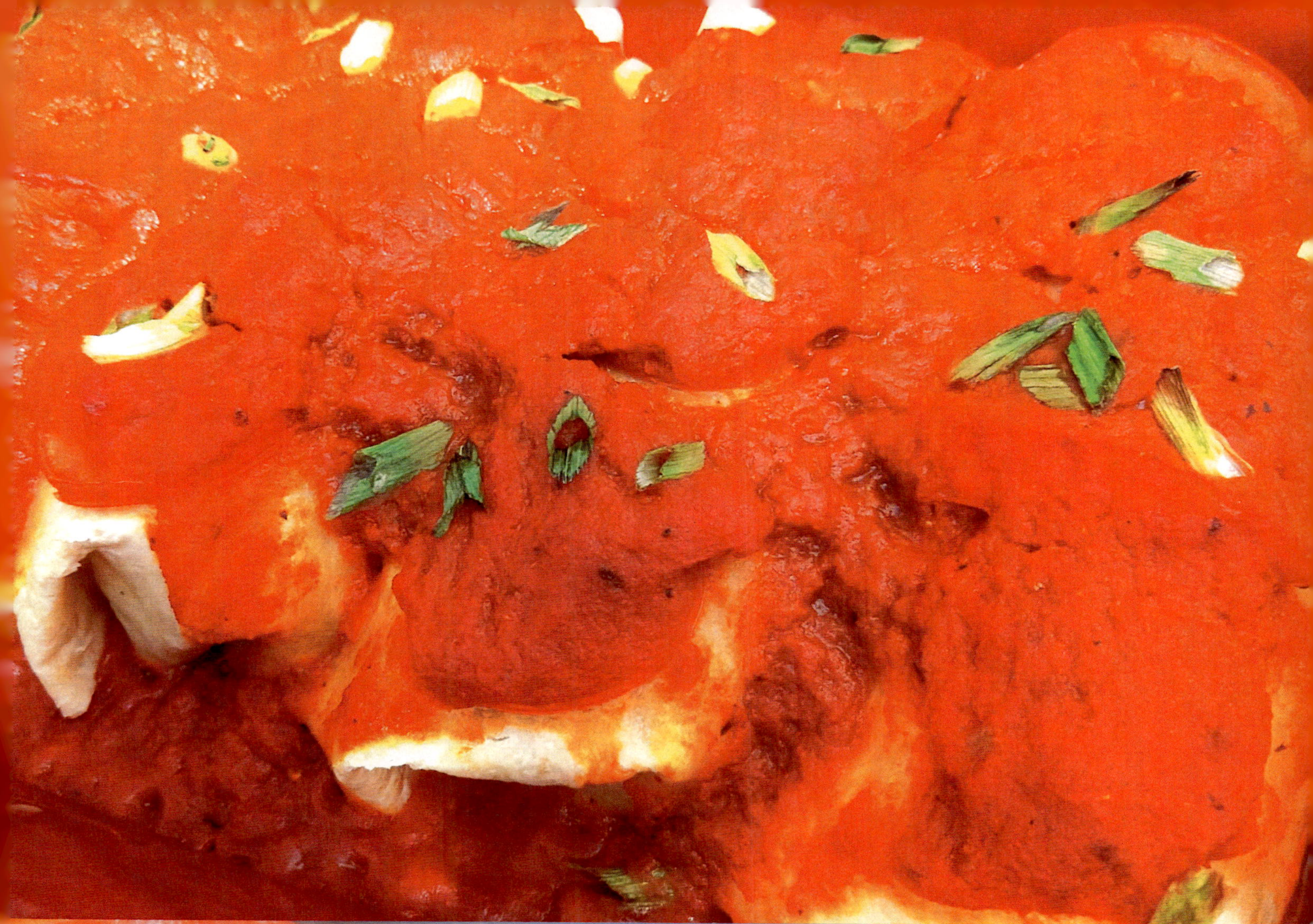

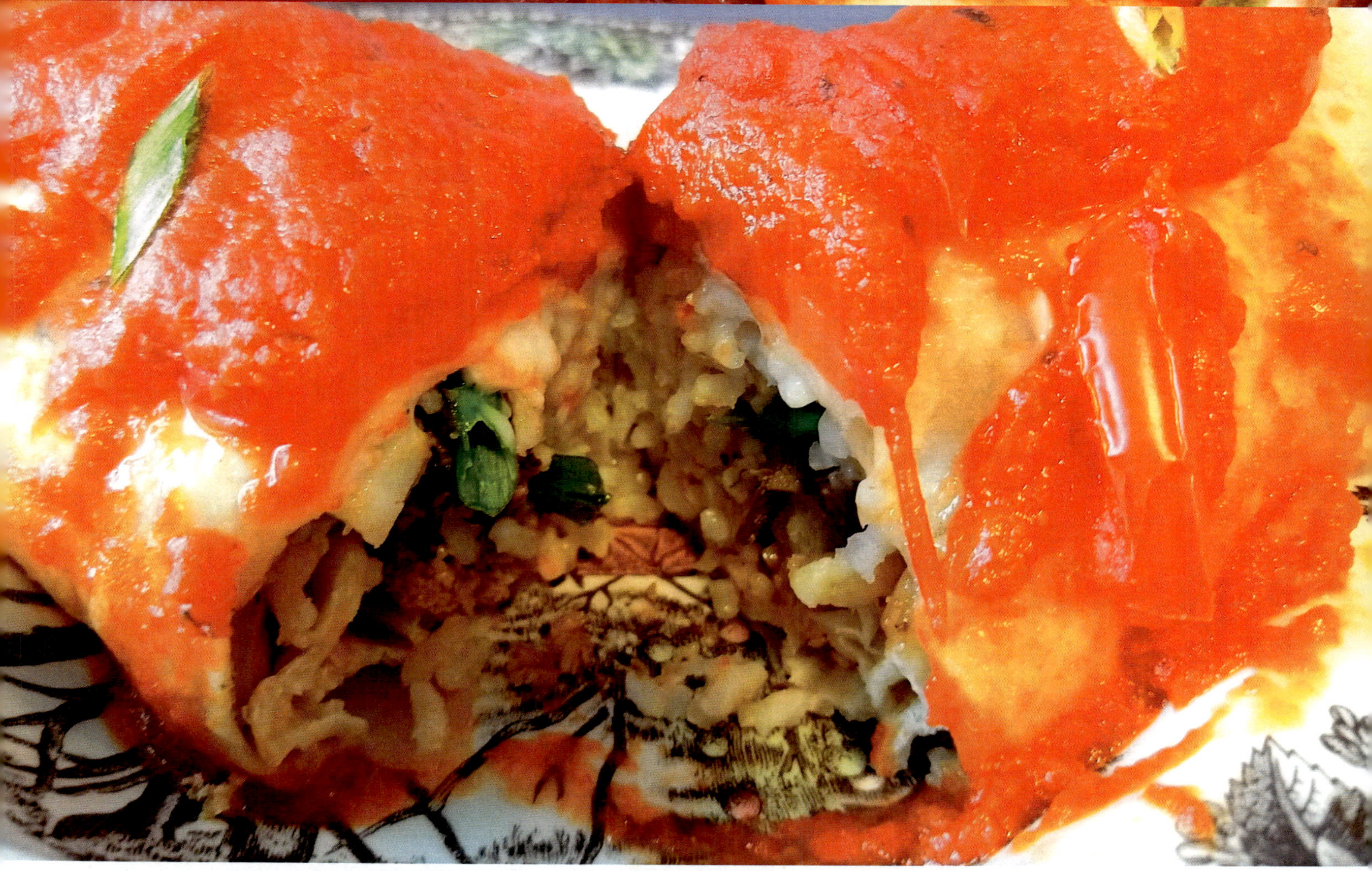

Cheater Peanut Sauce Pasta

serves 2

- 8 oz spaghetti, angel hair, ramen, or soba noodles, cooked (see notes)

CHEATER PEANUT SAUCE:

- 1/2 cup peanut butter
- 1/4 cup soy sauce
- 1/4 cup agave
- 1/4 water
- salt and pepper to taste (optional)
- Sriracha to taste (optional)

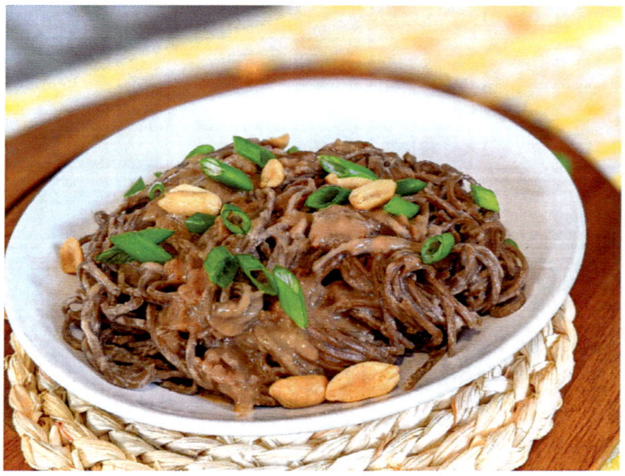

OPTIONAL TOPPINGS:

- sliced scallions
- tofu cubes
- peanuts
- edamame
- steamed greens
- frozen stir fry veggies, heated
- chopped cilantro

In a medium-sized microwave safe dish, add peanut sauce ingredients. Microwave for 30-60 seconds until you can easily stir/whisk with a fork until well blended. You can adjust the ratios to make it saltier (more soy sauce), sweeter (more agave), thinner (more water), or thicker (more peanut butter).

Pour over cooked pasta, add any optional toppings, and enjoy!

NOTES: This peanut sauce is also great as a dressing for a chopped salad or grain bowl (see Elevated Ramen on page 58). If you want to create a Thai-style peanut sauce, add a few tablespoons of coconut milk or coconut cream (optional: 1 TBSP tomato paste).

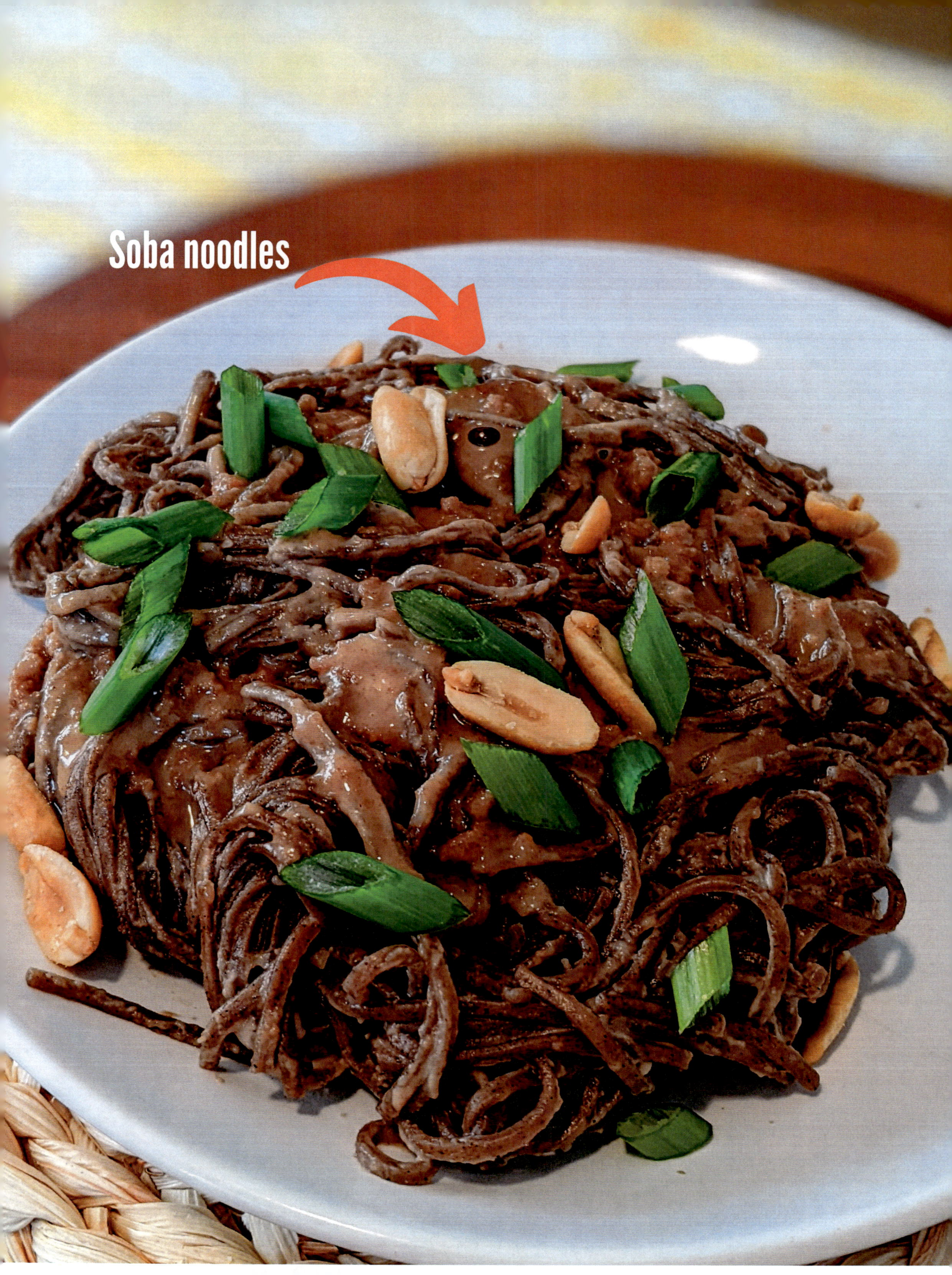
Soba noodles

Creamy Pumpkin Soup

serves 2

- 1 15-ounce can pureed pumpkin
- 1 13.5-ounce can full-fat, unsweetened coconut milk
- Salt and pepper to taste

In a microwave safe dish, combine ingredients and microwave for about 60 seconds and stir. Continue microwaving until desired temperature is reached.

Enjoy as is, or over pasta or rice. You can also add vegan sausage, sundried tomatoes, and/or beans to turn this into a scrumptious and filling stew!

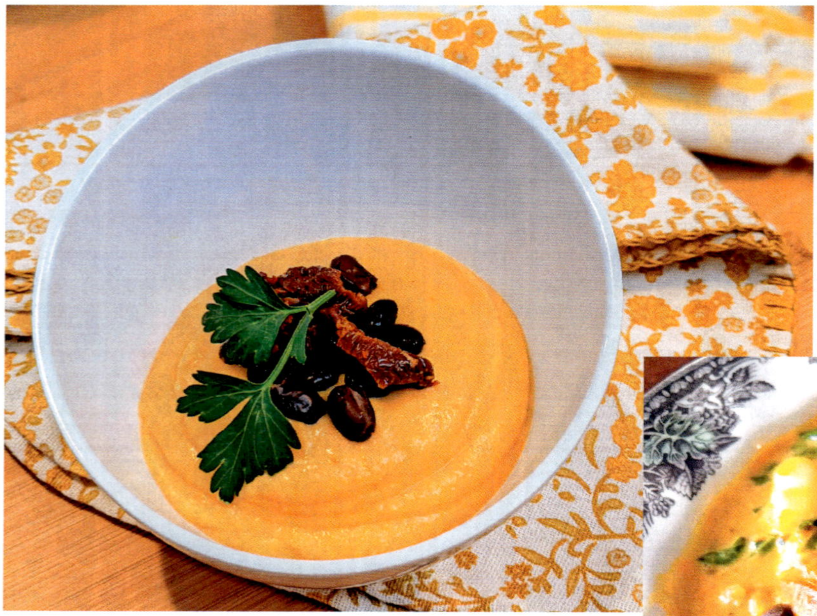

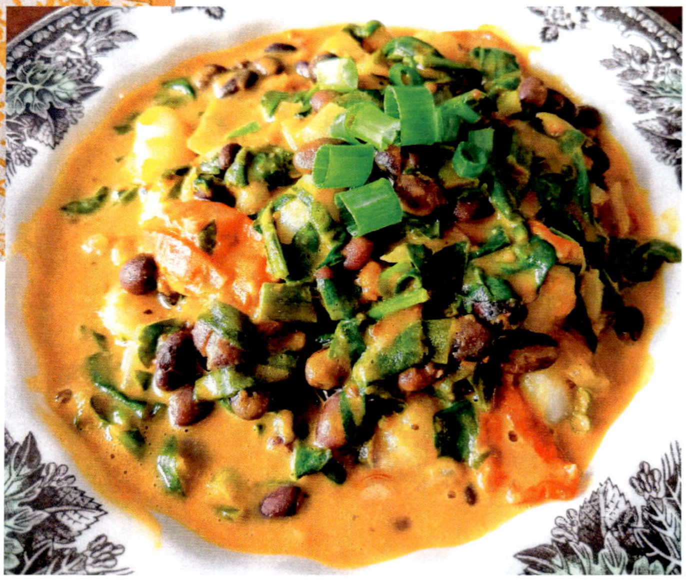

Creamy Tomato Soup and Rice

Needs Stovetop / Hot plate

serves 2

- 1 13.5-ounce can full-fat, unsweetened coconut milk
- 1 15-oz can plain tomato sauce
- 1/2 cup of your favorite rice
- 1 cup water
- Salt and pepper to taste

For best results, you'll need a hot plate or stovetop for this recipe. In a small saucepan, combine all ingredients and bring to a simmer. To figure out how long to simmer, check your rice package instructions. Short grain white rice (e.g., jasmine) should simmer for 15 minutes and rest for 10. Long grain brown rice (e.g., basmati) should simmer for 40 minutes and rest for 10.

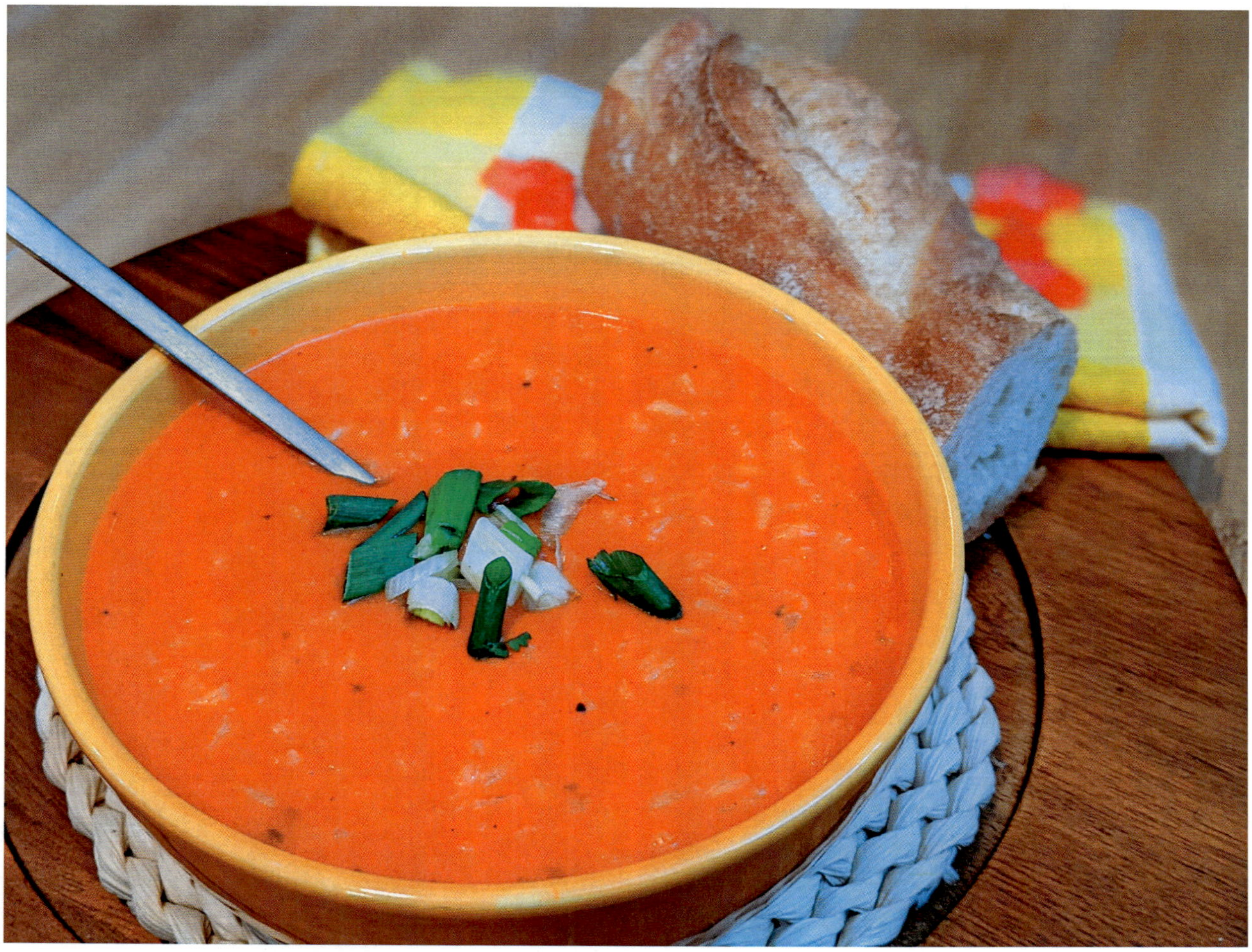

Elevated Ramen

serves 1

- 1 package (3.5 oz) ramen noodles (see notes)
- Enough water to cover noodles (1-2 cups)
- Sliced scallions for topping (optional)

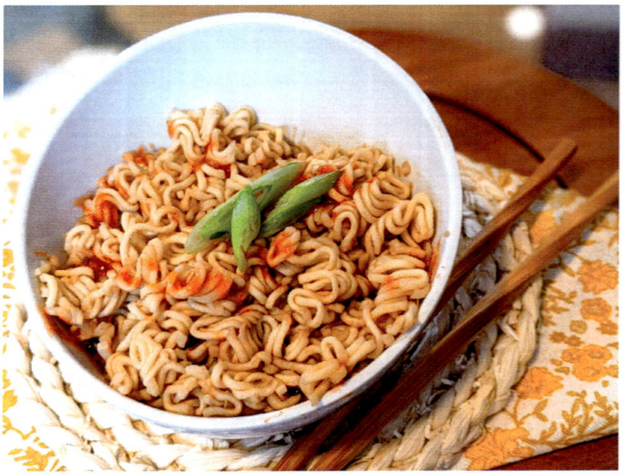

Elevated Sauce:

- 1/3 cup soy sauce
- 1/3 cup water
- 2 TBSP agave
- 2 TBSP rice vinegar
- 1 teaspoon minced garlic or garlic powder
- 1 teaspoon minced ginger or ginger powder
- 2 teaspoons sriracha or other hot sauce (optional)

In a microwave safe container, crumble one package ramen noodles and cover with water. Place the lid loosely on top and microwave on high for two minutes (you may need to adjust cook time slightly to cook noodles to your liking).

While ramen is microwaving, combine all Elevated Sauce ingredients in a bowl/small container and whisk with a fork.

Strain noodles (if you have a microwave container with a steam valve, you can pour water out through this!) and pour your Elevated Sauce over top. If you want it piping hot, you can return the cooked noodles and sauce to the microwave for another 30 seconds.

Top with sliced scallions (if using) and dig in!

NOTES: We love this sauce because it doesn't have any scary ramen packet ingredients (e.g., MSG) in it. The noodles usually aren't all-natural either, so if you prefer, you can use this Elevated Sauce on any other kind of noodle (e.g., soba, rice, angel hair, etc.)!

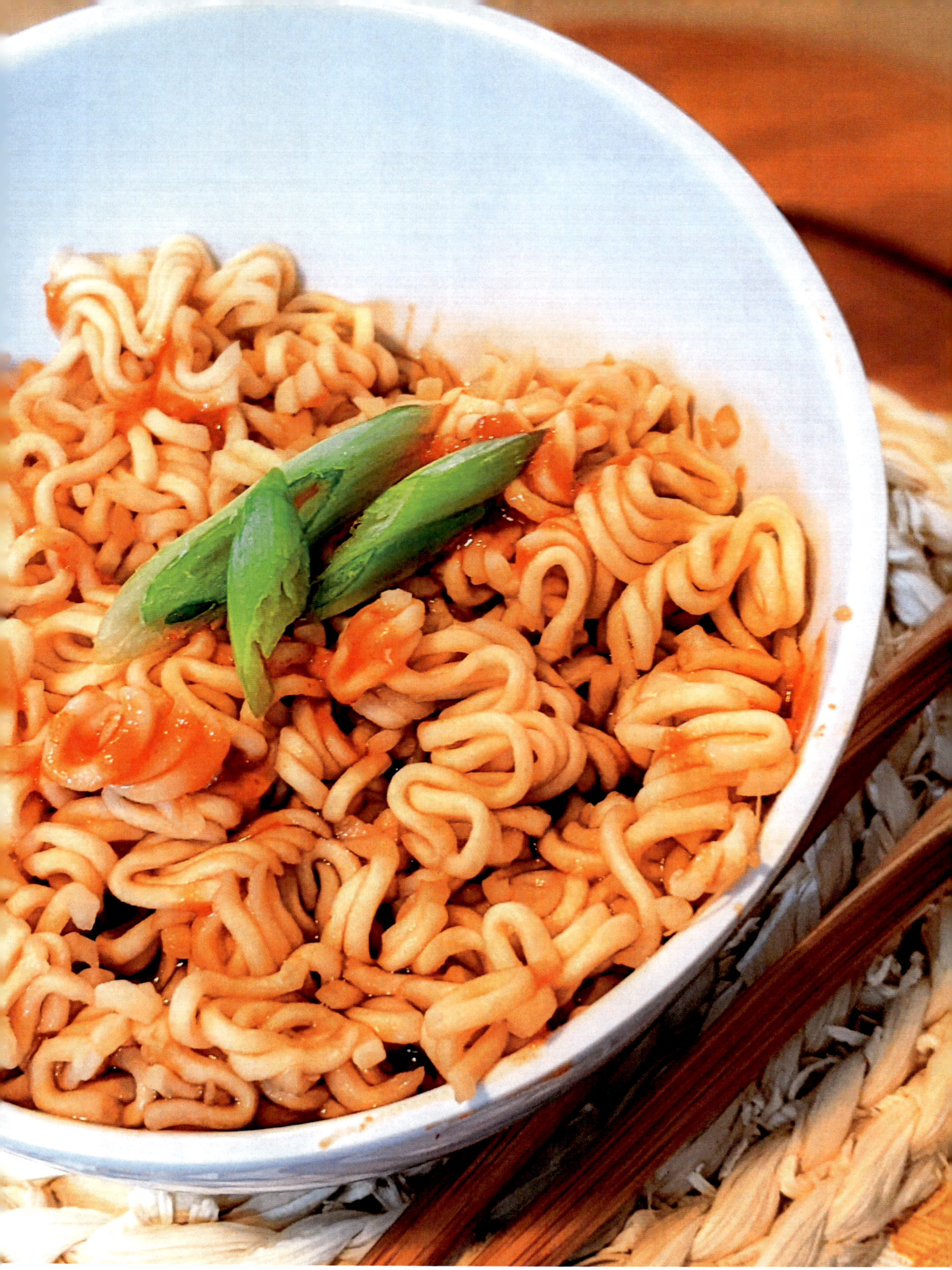

Falafel Wrap

serves 1

- 1 burrito-sized tortilla
- 3-4 frozen falafel, heated
- 1/4 cucumber, sliced or chopped
- 1 /2 plum tomato, sliced or chopped (optional)
- fresh parsley or scallions, chopped (optional)
- 1/4 cup vegan feta (optional)

FOR SPREAD (see notes):

- 3 TBSP vegan sour cream or cream cheese
- 1/2 TBSP dried dill

Make spread by softening cream cheese in the microwave for about 20 seconds (not necessary if using vegan sour cream) and stir in dried dill. Spread across tortilla and layer the rest of your ingredients. Roll up (see page 40 for tortilla-rolling tips) and dig in!

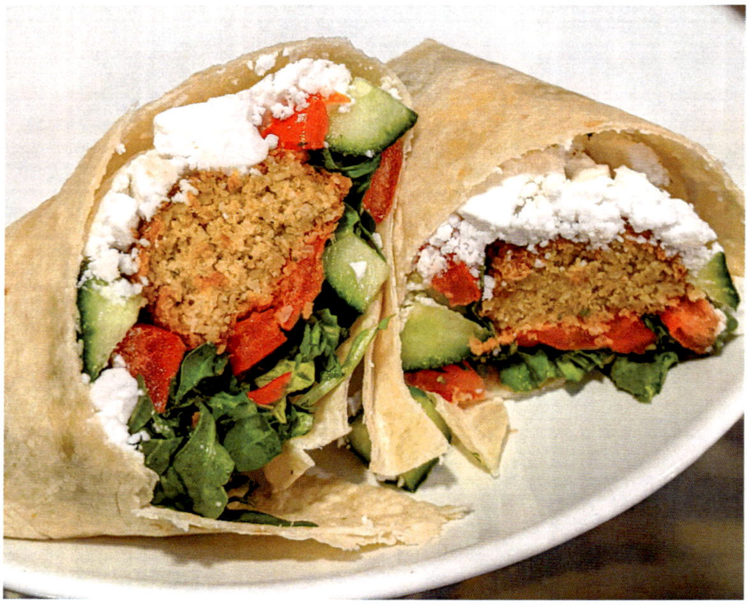

NOTES: For best results, make spread 4+ hours ahead and refrigerate (overnight is best). Tahini or plain vegan yogurt also make great additions if your wrap is too dry.

Gnocchi with Sundried Tomatoes

Needs Stovetop / Hot plate

serves 2

- 1 package (17-18 oz) gnocchi (check to make sure it doesn't contain eggs) -OR- orzo pasta
- 1 jar (8-9 oz) chopped or julienned sundried tomatoes packed in oil
- 1 package (6-8 oz) spinach (optional)
- Salt and pepper to taste

OPTIONAL TOPPINGS:

- Vegan parmesan cheese
- Nutritional yeast
- Crushed nuts
- Vegan sausage

In a medium sized pot, boil gnocchi according to package instructions. Strain and return to stovetop/hot plate. Pour in jar of sundried tomatoes (and spinach, if using). Stir until spinach wilts (if applicable). Add salt and pepper (and any optional toppings) to taste.

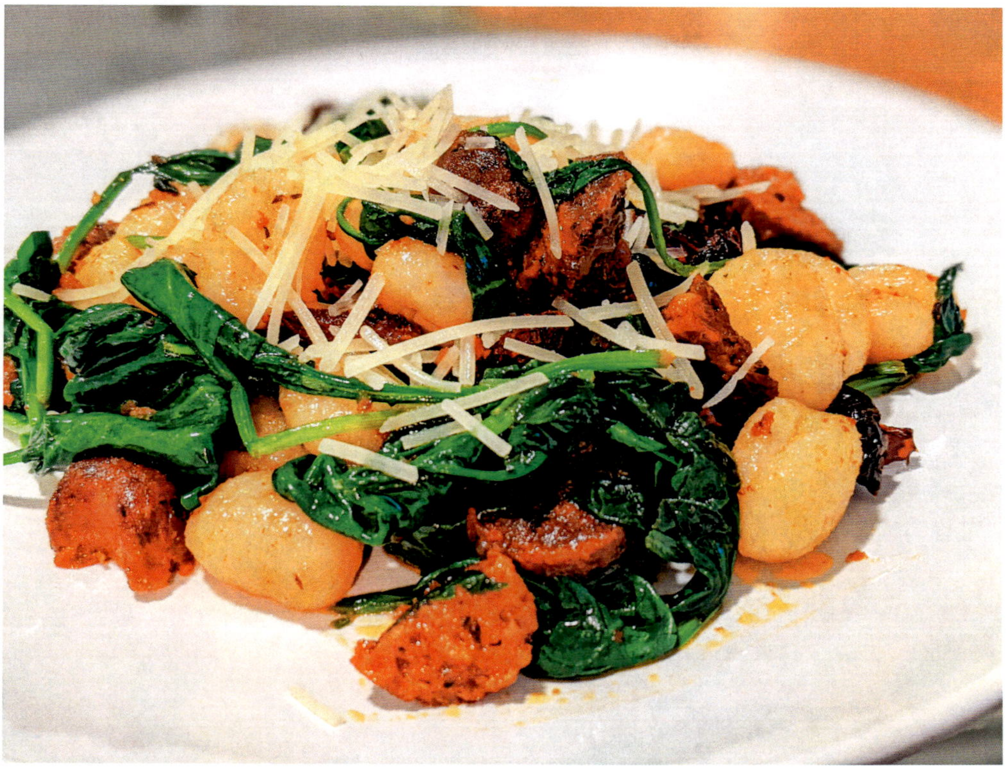

Loaded Sweet Potato

serves 1

- 1 large sweet potato
- 1/2 cup black beans
- 1/2 cup steamed greens, e.g., spinach, kale, collards (see instructions)
- Salt and pepper to taste

OPTIONAL TOPPINGS:

- Vegan cheese
- Nutritional yeast
- Vegan butter
- Vegan salad dressing (see page 32)

Prick sweet potato several times with a fork and place in a large microwave safe dish with a lid loosely over top. Microwave on high for 6 minutes. If the sweet potato is especially large, it might take about 8 minutes to cook through. (To roast in the oven: prick with fork, place on foil or baking sheet, and bake for one hour at 425 degrees Fahrenheit.)

While sweet potato is cooking, rinse and strain black beans (see page 11 for straining tips).

Once the sweet potato is cooked through, keep it in the microwave container and slice it open. Dump a large handful of greens on top. Place the lid loosely back on the container and microwave for another 20-30 seconds or until greens are wilted.

Lastly, add beans and any other optional toppings and dive it!

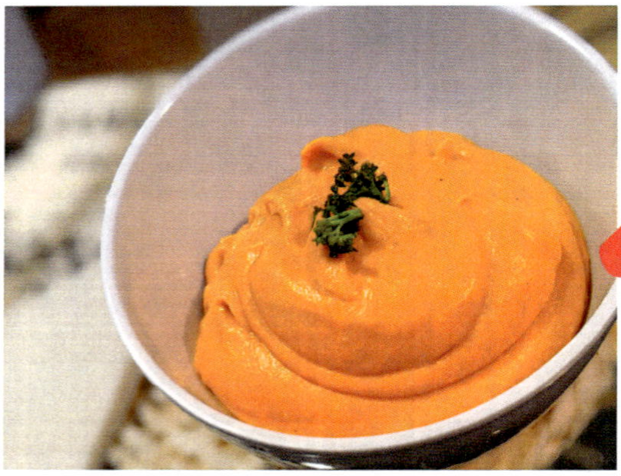

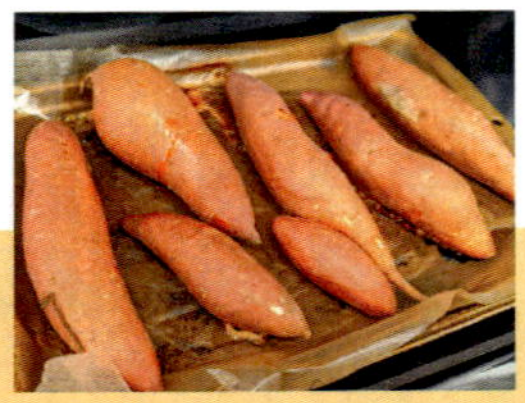

Calling all chefs

If you have access to an oven and food processor or beaters, you can make our Savory Whipped Sweet Potatoes! (Recipe video on YouTube!)

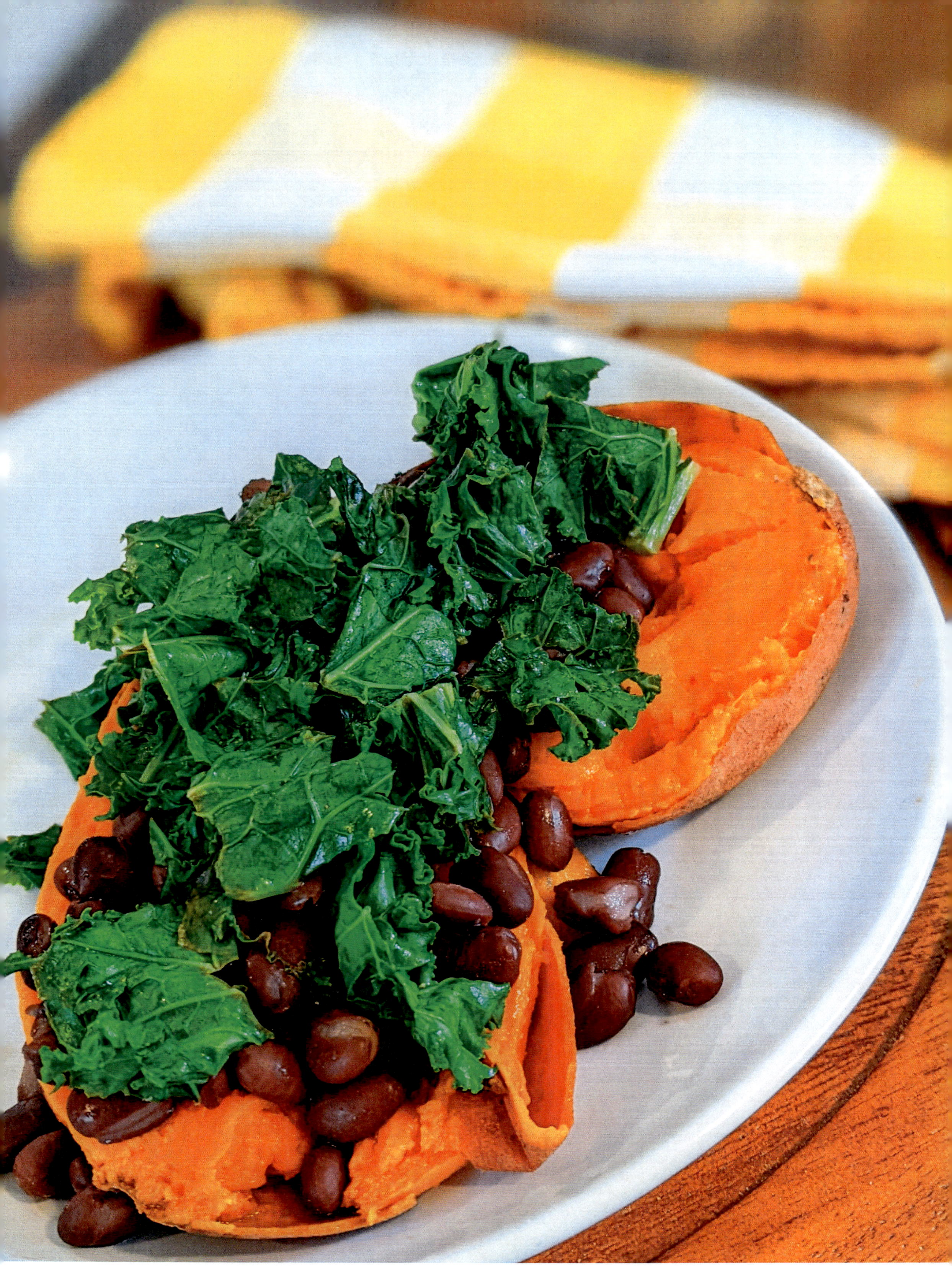

Oatmeal Bowls

serves 1

Base:

- 1/2 cup oats
- 1 cup water

Combine in a microwave safe dish and microwave for 1 minute and 20 seconds. Then add the ingredients from your chosen flavor combo:

Sweet PB+J:

  - 1 large scoop of nut butter (peanut, almond, cashew)
  - 1 large scoop scoop of jelly (flavor of choice)
  - Handful of coconut shreds, crushed peanuts and/or chocolate chips

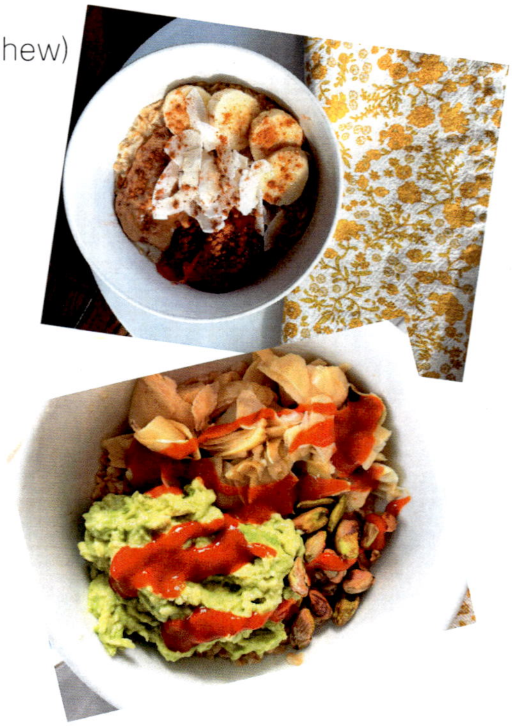

Savory Artichoke + Avocado:

  - 1-2 mashed avocados
  - Handful of pistachios (shelled)
  - Small portion of roughly chopped artichokes, rinsed and drained from a can
  - Drizzle of sriracha or hot sauce (optional)

Snacky Oats:

- BBQ Chickpea Salad (page 50)
- 1 avocado, sliced or mashed
- Drizzle of BBQ sauce

Hearty Oats:

- Any extra fruit from your fridge
- Drizzle of maple syrup or agave
- Handful of nuts (cashews, peanuts, almonds)

Overnight Oats

serves 2-3

- 1 cup rolled oats
- 1 cup non-dairy milk
- ¼ cup almond or peanut butter
- 1 teaspoon cinnamon
- ¼ cup sliced strawberries or your favorite fruit (can use frozen)
- 1 tablespoon nuts (your choice), chopped
- Pinch of salt and vanilla (optional)

Combine all ingredients in a medium-sized container and stir. Put lid on and place in fridge overnight. Can be warmed up in the morning if you prefer!

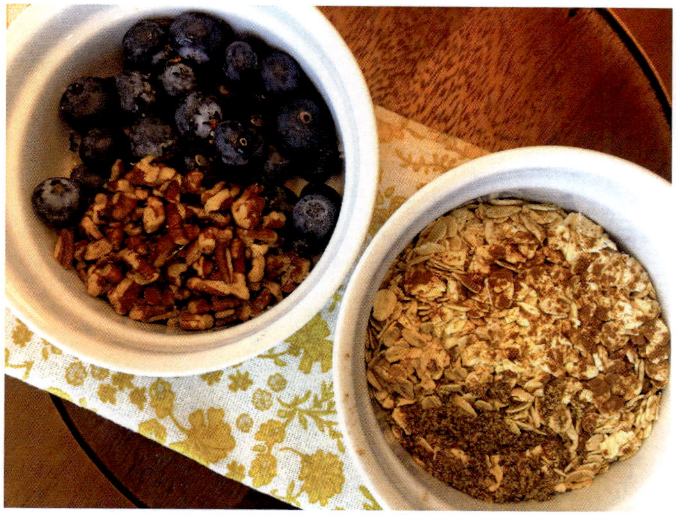

Let's talk about oats!

So simple. So inexpensive. They're gluten-free, super nutritious, and something you can add into your meal planning any time of day. Oats are also a complex carbohydrate that fuels your mind, body + soul. These magical little grains will also contribute to a swift burst of serotonin to keep you going on those long nights out, we mean, late nights in the library.

NOTES: Maple syrup, agave, and/or dried fruit make wonderful additions.

Needs Stovetop / Hot plate

Panini Paradise

serves 1

- 2 slices of your favorite bread (white, wheat, rye, baguette, etc.)
- 2 slices (or 1/2 cup shreds) of your favorite vegan cheese
- 2-3 TBSP vegan butter or mayo

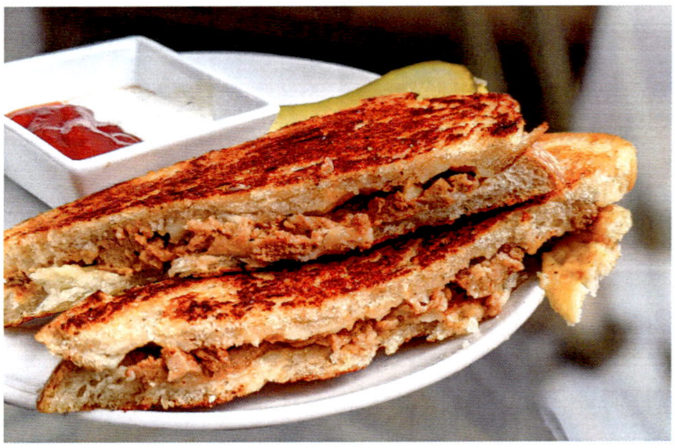

FILLING OPTIONS:

- Pickle sandwich slices
- Vegan ham, turkey, tofu, or bacon slices
- Sliced avocado
- Tomato slices
- Steamed greens
- Sauerkraut
- Pickled peppers
- Your favorite condiment/dressing (spread on the inside)
- [insert your creative idea here!]

On stovetop or hot plate, heat a small frying pan to medium heat. Generously spread vegan butter or mayo on one side of each slice of bread. Place the first slice, butter/mayo side down, in the heated frying pan. Put one slice (or 1/4 cup shreds) of cheese on top of bread. Layer your filling options on top of cheese and place the second slice (or 1/4 cup shreds) of cheese on top. Lastly, place the second piece of bread on your delicious stack, butter/mayo side facing up.

Using a spatula (or other flipping tool), press firmly down on the panini for several seconds. Check regularly; the first side should be a perfect golden brown after a few minutes. Flip, and again press the sandwich down for several seconds using your spatula. (This will give your sandwich the panini press crunch!)

Once it's golden brown on both sides, remove from pan and slice on the diagonal (if you're feelin' fancy)!.

NOTES: Keeping the pan at a lower (medium) heat and pressing sandwich into pan will ensure a deep, golden brown crunch. Cooking at a higher temperature is faster, but results aren't as crunchy!

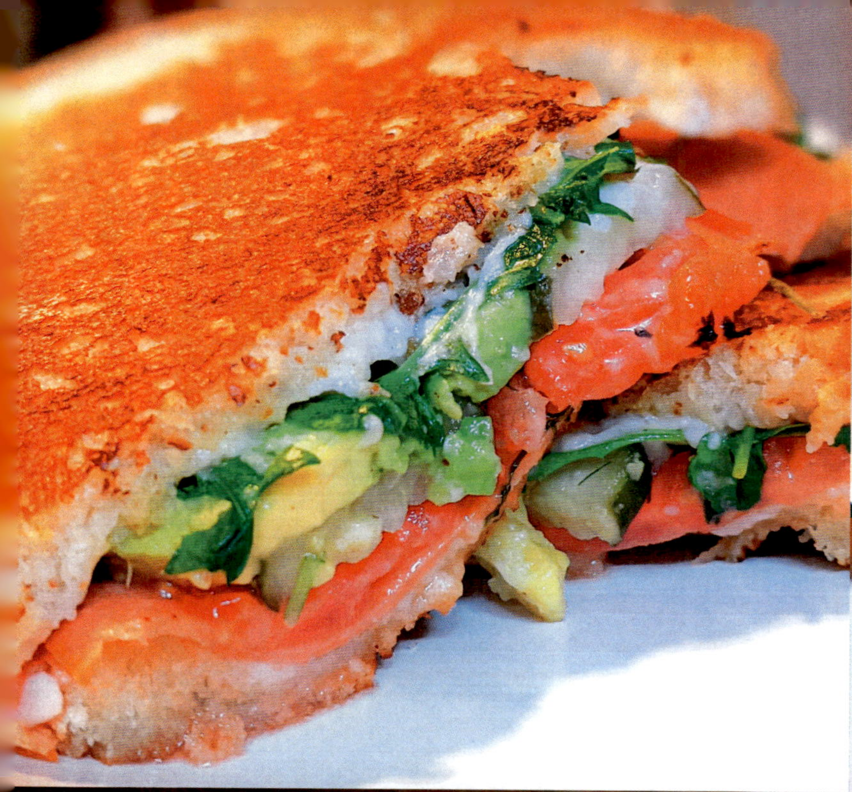
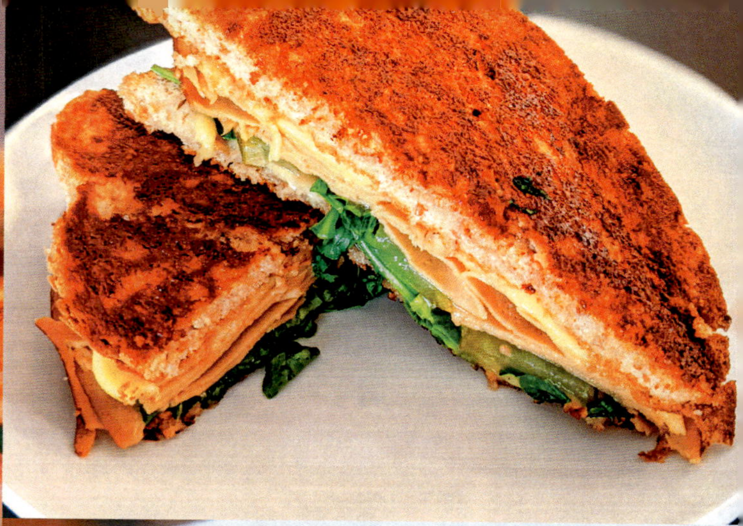
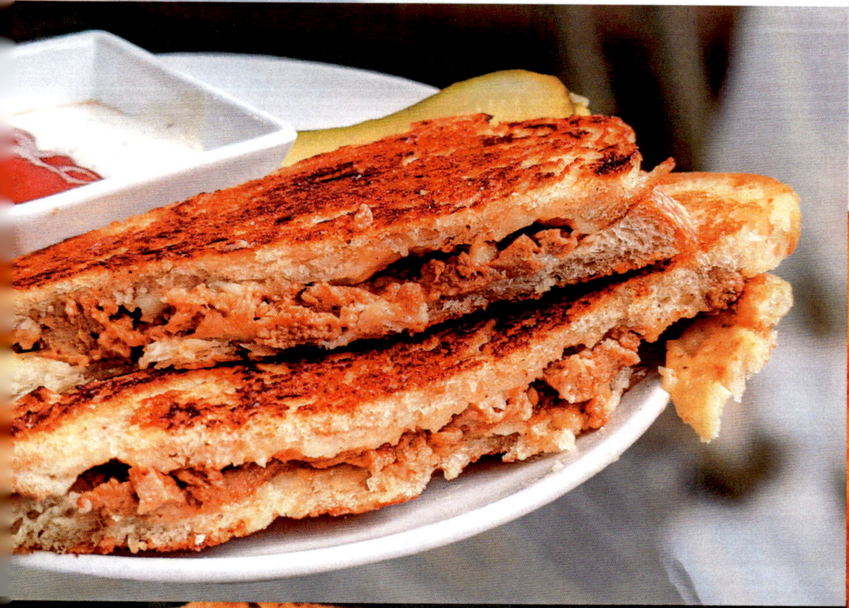
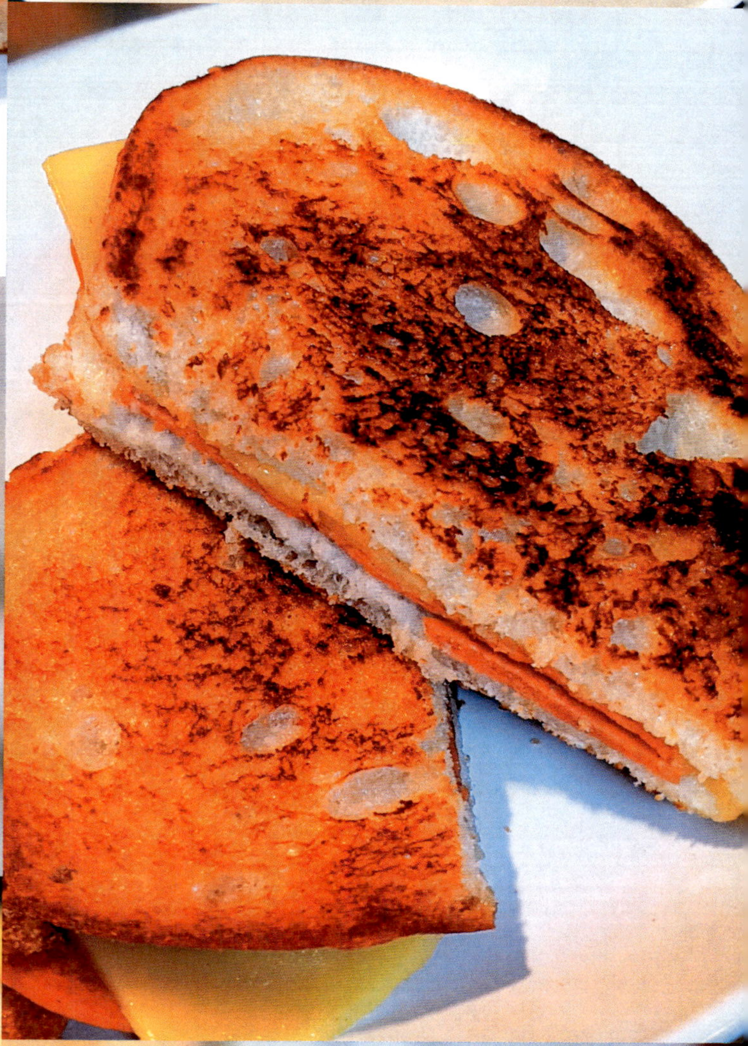
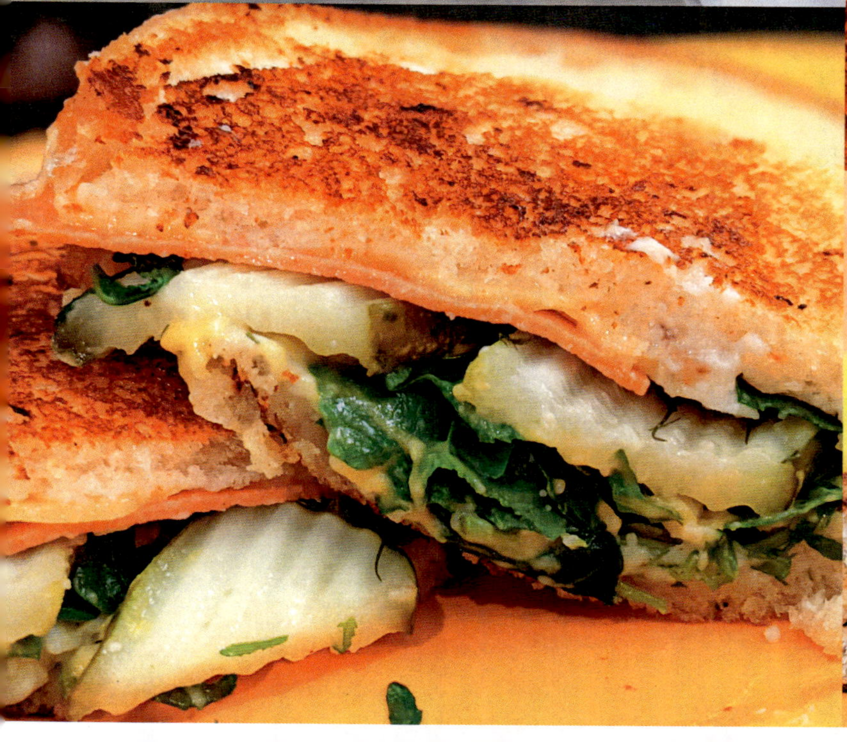
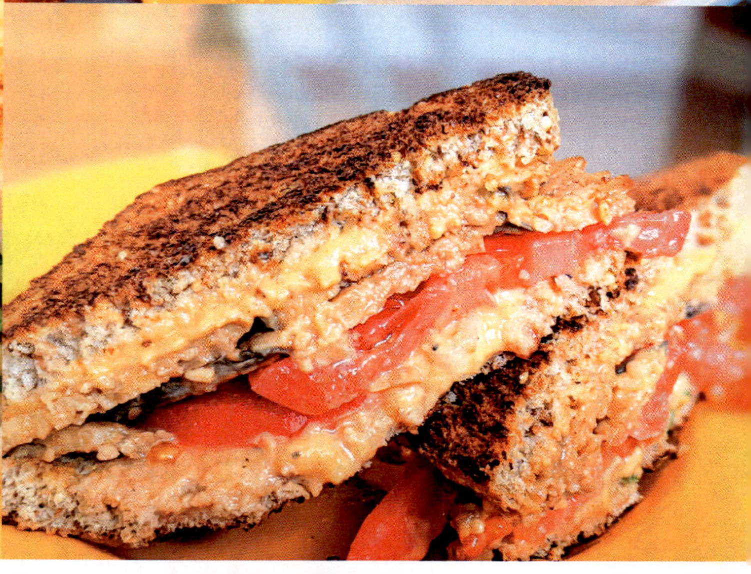

Pita Pizza

Needs Oven / Toaster oven

serves 1

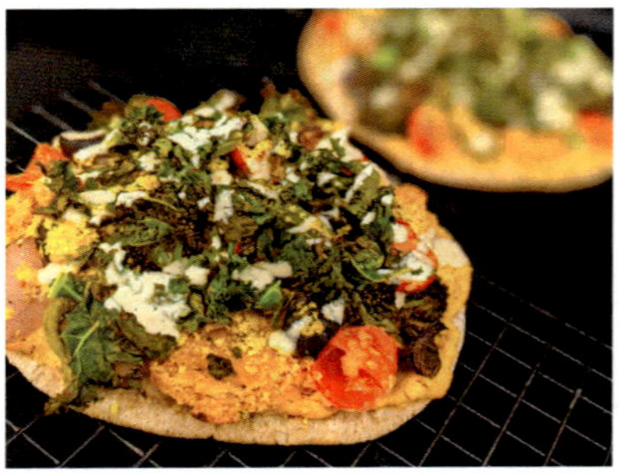

- 1 pita

SAUCE/SPREAD OPTIONS:

- Hummus
- Refried beans
- Tomato sauce
- Vegan cream cheese (note: this can get a little too 'melty')
- [insert your creative idea here!]

TOPPING OPTIONS:

- Vegan cheese or nutritional yeast
- Sliced veggies (onion, pepper, tomato, olive, broccoli, zucchini, etc.)
- Your favorite vegan meat (sausage, pepperoni, bacon, chick'n, etc.)
- Pickled/hot peppers
- [insert your creative idea here!]

FINAL TOUCHES (OPTIONAL):

- Arugula
- Avocado
- Drizzled mustard, dressing, or your favorite condiment
- Fresh chopped herbs (basil, cilantro, parsley, scallions, etc.)

Preheat oven/toaster oven to 375 degrees Fahrenheit. Evenly spread a layer of "sauce" on top of your pita and arrange toppings over sauce.

Place directly on oven rack and bake for 10 minutes. Add any final touches if using. Let cool for a minute or two, slice and enjoy!

NOTES: Almost anything will work here if you stick to a theme! We've even used leftover Indian take-out to make an Indian themed pita pizza! (Pictured middle right on next page.)

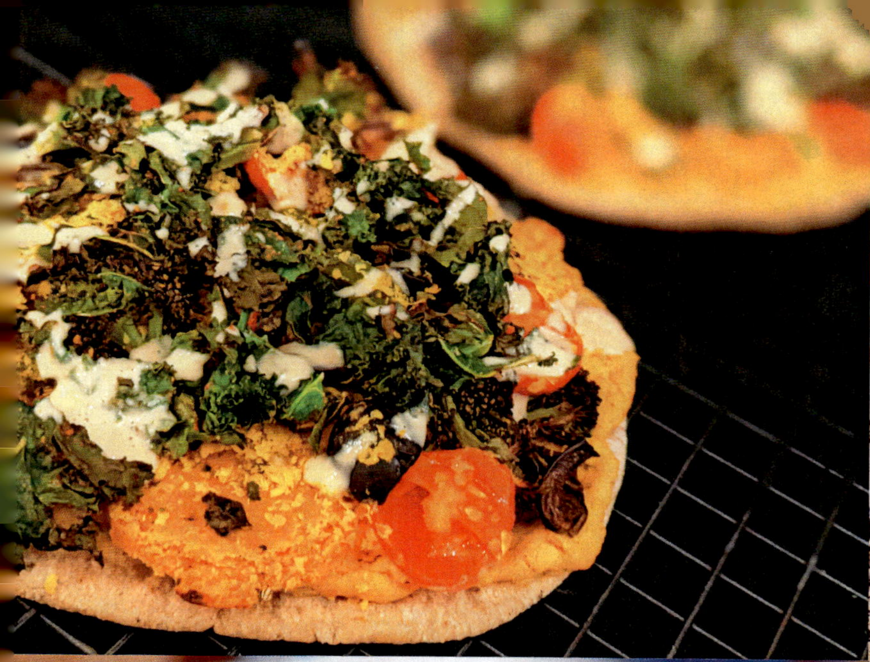
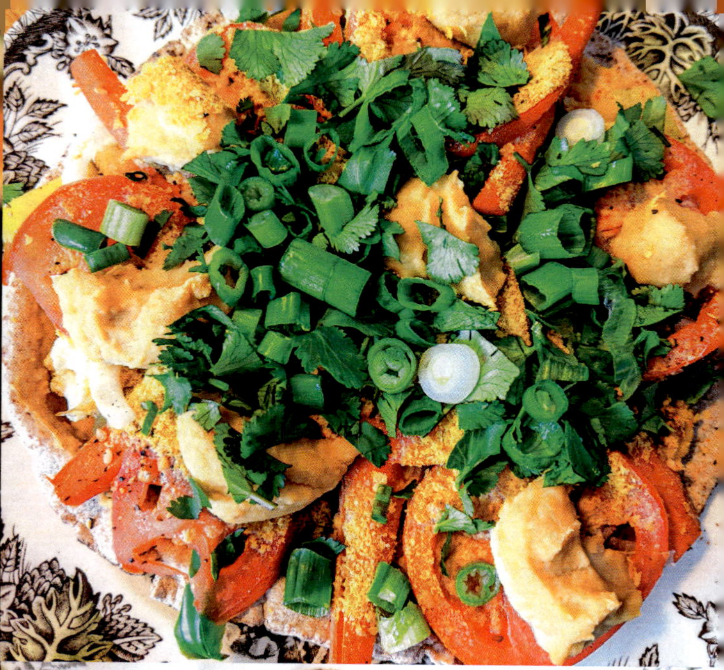
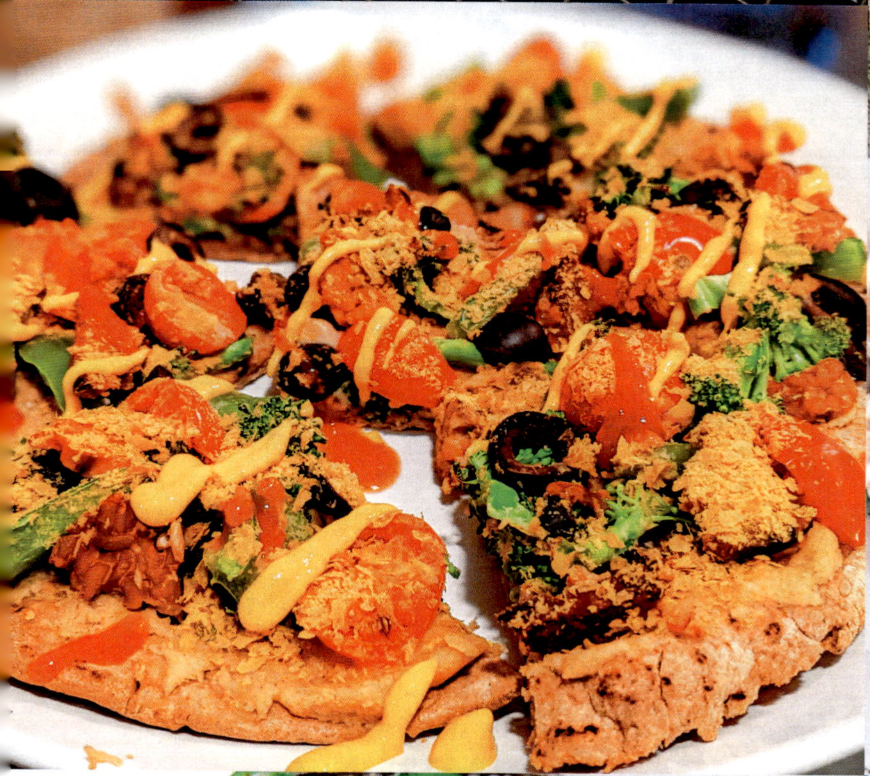
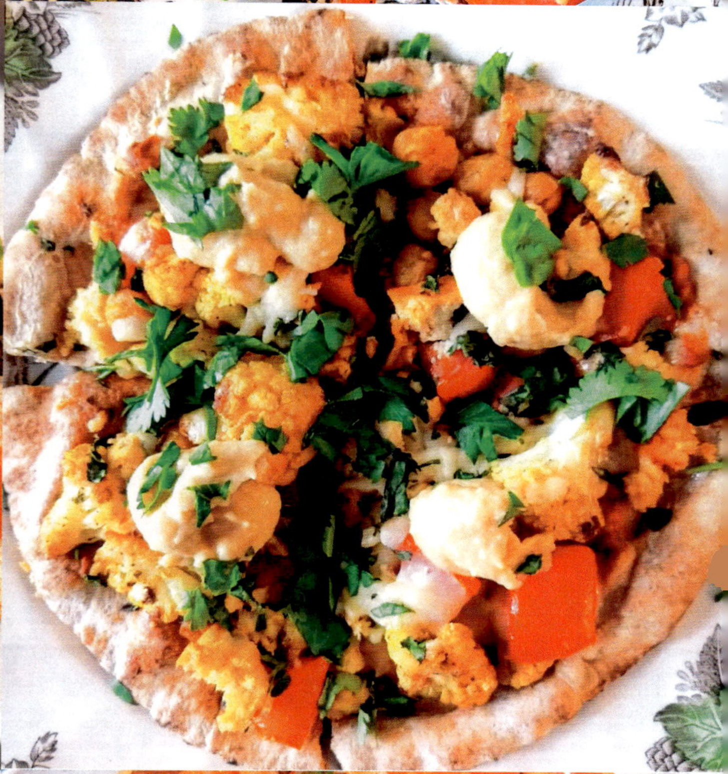
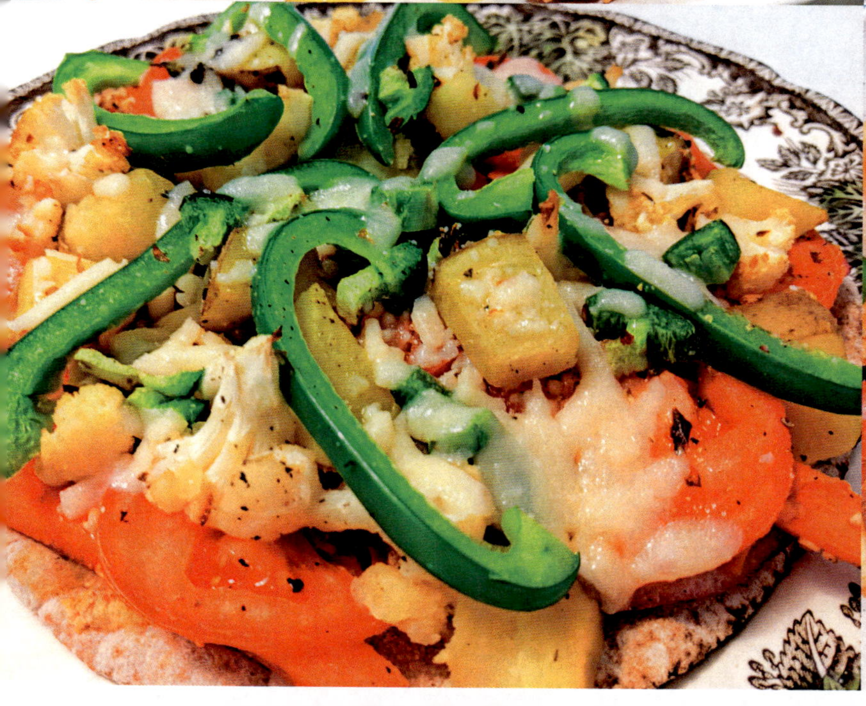
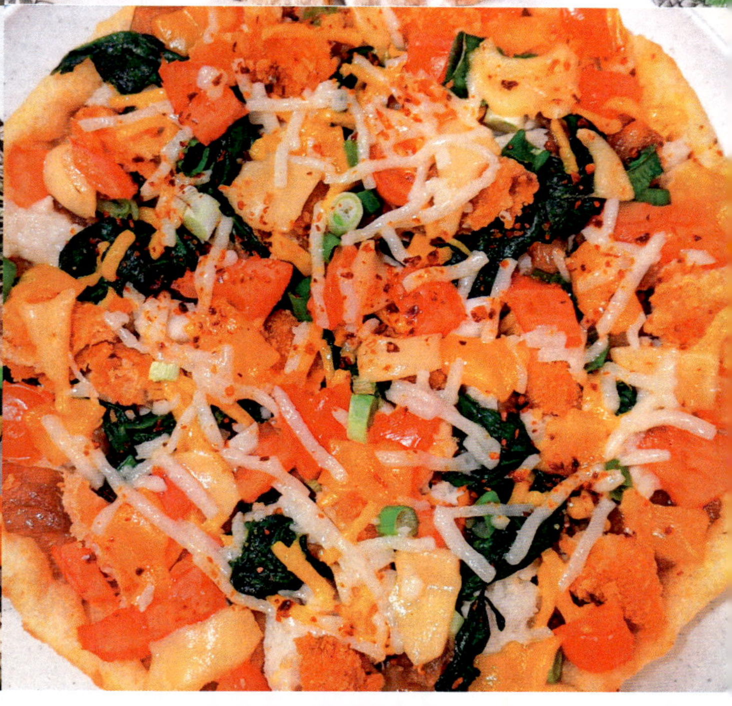

Polenta with Chili + Greens

serves 2

- 4 polenta slices (see notes)
- 1 can vegetarian/vegan chili (can substitute baked beans)
- 2-3 cups greens (spinach, kale, collards, etc.)
- Nutritional yeast or vegan cheese for topping (optional)

In a large microwave safe dish, place polenta slices on the bottom. Pour chili over top. Microwave for 2-3 minutes or until it's hot and bubbling. Add greens and loosely place lid on top.. Microwave for an additional 20-30 seconds or until greens are wilted. Top with nutritional yeast or vegan cheese (if using) and dig in!

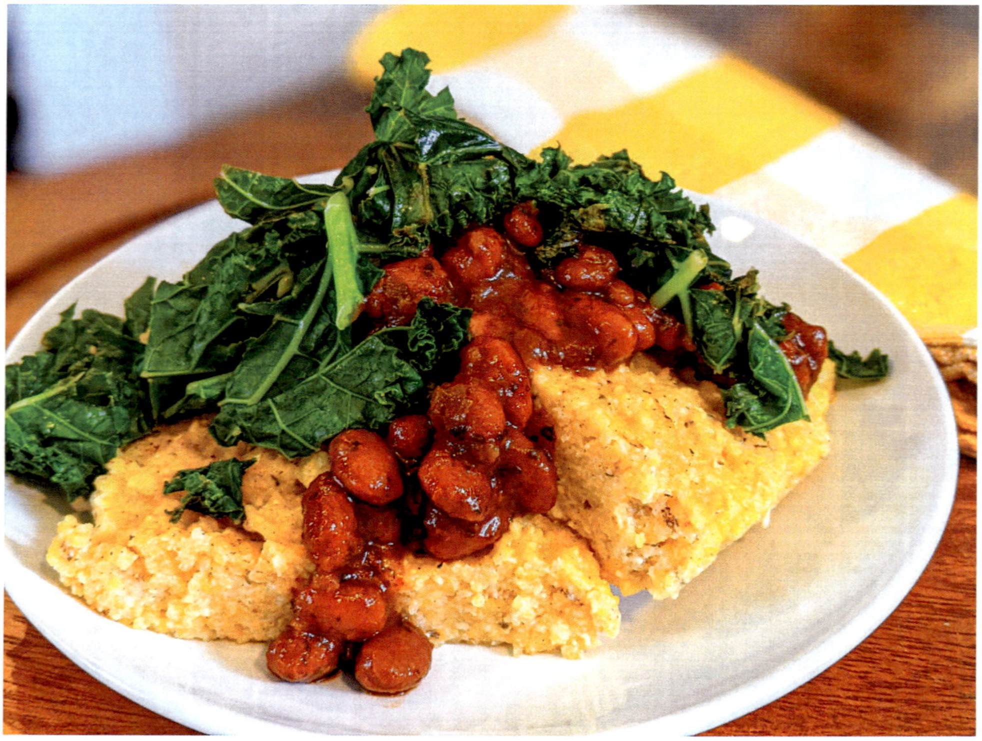

NOTES: In some stores, you can purchase cooked polenta in a tube that's ready to slice and eat (sold near the pasta; not refrigerated). Otherwise, if you have a stovetop, you can purchase corn grits (sold near flour and baking goods) and prepare according to package instructions, which is also cheap and delicious! If you want to go the extra mile, try frying the polenta slices before eating!

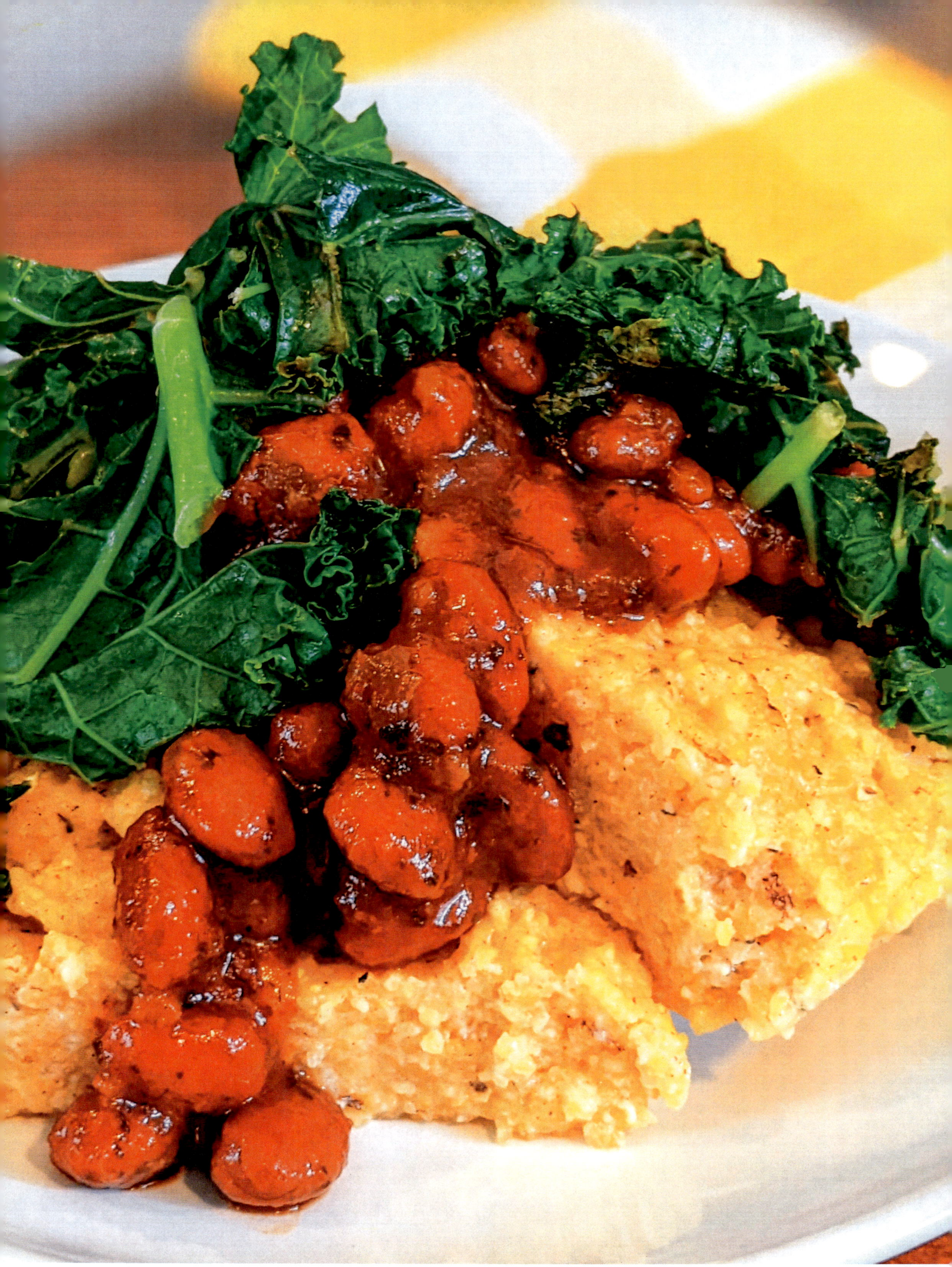

Quick Quesdilla

Needs Stovetop / Hot plate

serves 1

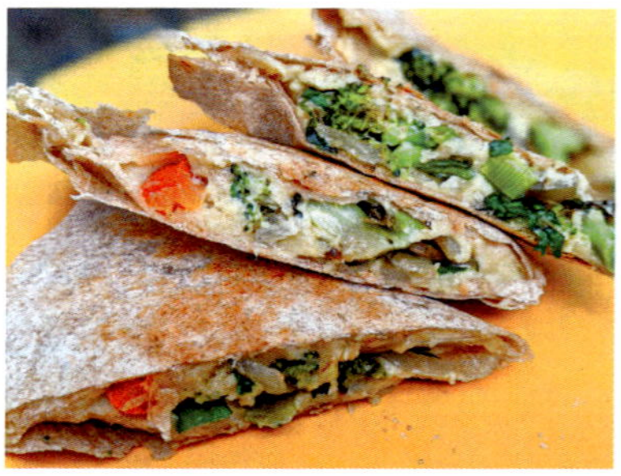

- 1 burrito-sized tortilla

SAUCE/SPREAD OPTIONS:

- Hummus
- Refried beans
- Tomato sauce
- Vegan cream cheese (note: this can get a little too 'melty')
- [insert your creative idea here!]

FILLING OPTIONS:

- Vegan cheese or nutritional yeast
- Sliced veggies (onion, pepper, tomato, olive, broccoli, zucchini, etc.)
- Your favorite vegan meat (soy chorizo, sausage, pepperoni, bacon, chick'n, etc.)
- Potato cubes or hash browns
- Avocado
- Sundried tomatoes

DIPPING OPTIONS:

- Ketchup or your favorite condiment
- Hot sauce, salsa, or tomato sauce
- Vegan sour cream
- Salad dressing (see page 32)

On stovetop or hot plate, heat a large frying pan to medium heat. Spread your sauce across the whole tortilla and fill one half of it with your chosen fillings. Fold tortilla half and place on heated pan. Toast on each side (a few minutes per side or until golden brown), then slice into 2-4 pieces with a sharp knife or pizza cutter and enjoy!

NOTES: Keeping the pan at a lower (medium) heat will ensure a deep, golden brown crunch. Cooking at a higher temperature is faster, but results aren't as crunchy! As with our pita pizzas and paninis, almost any fillings will work!

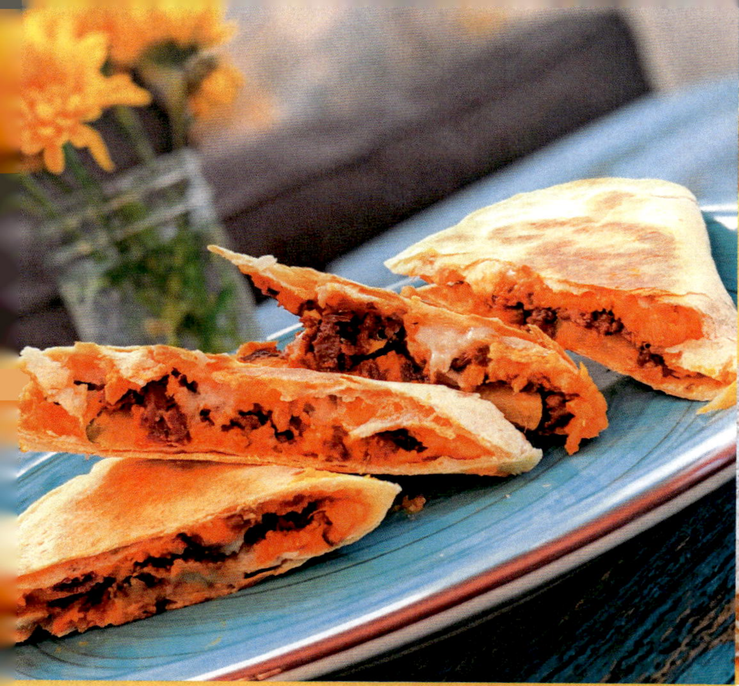
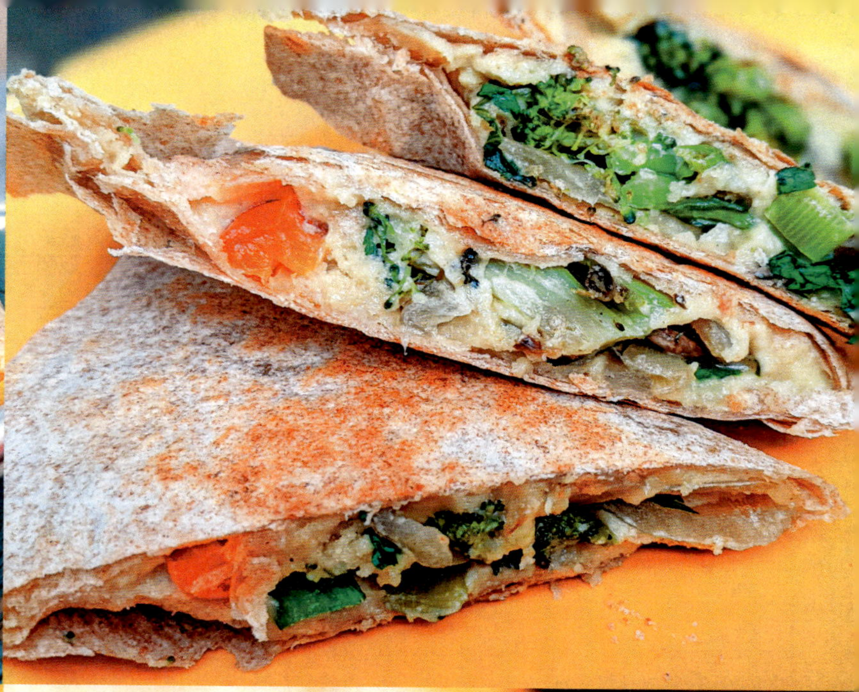
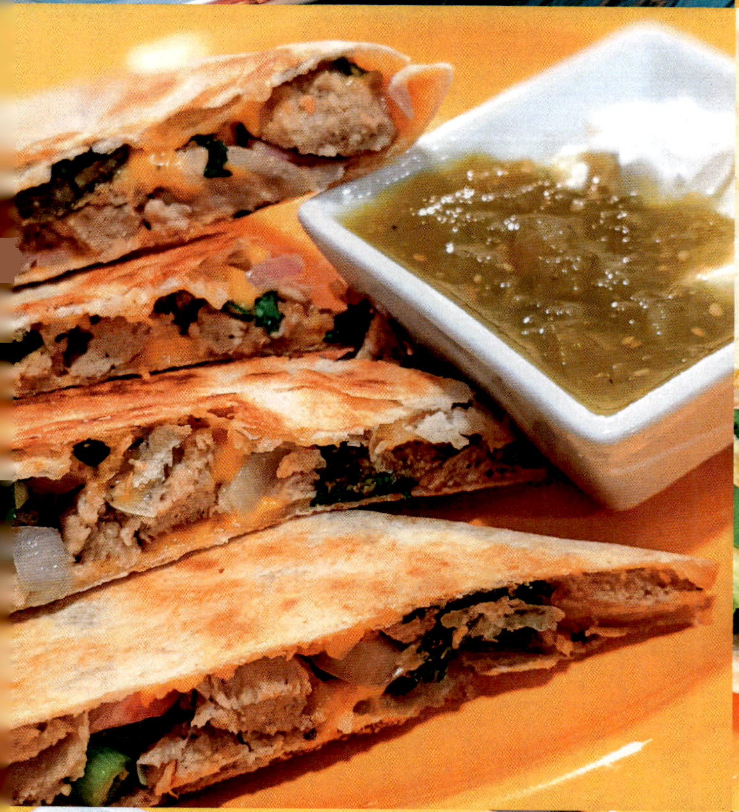
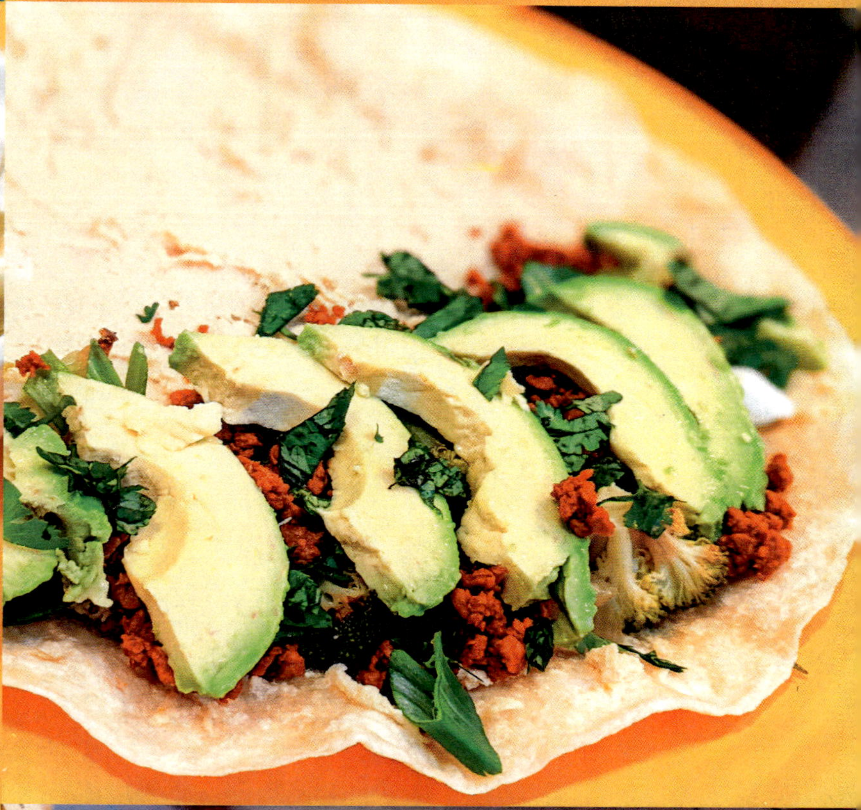
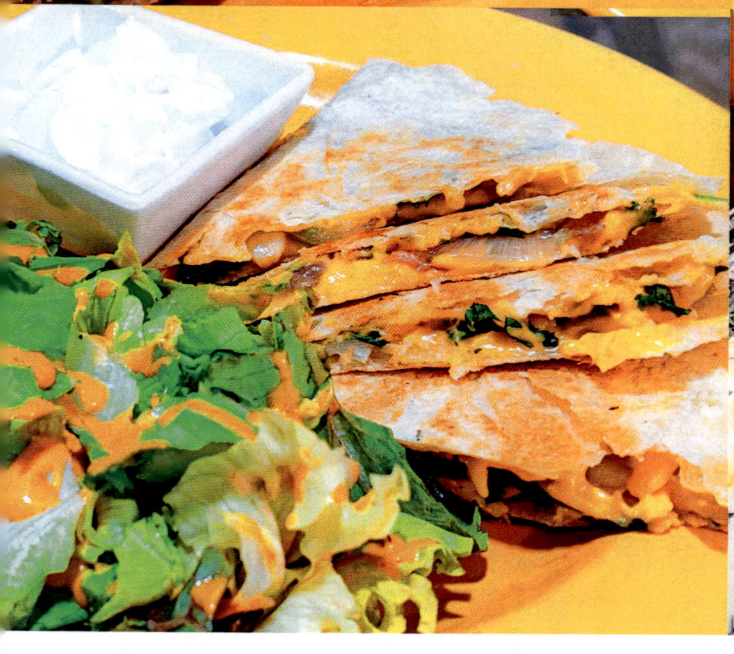
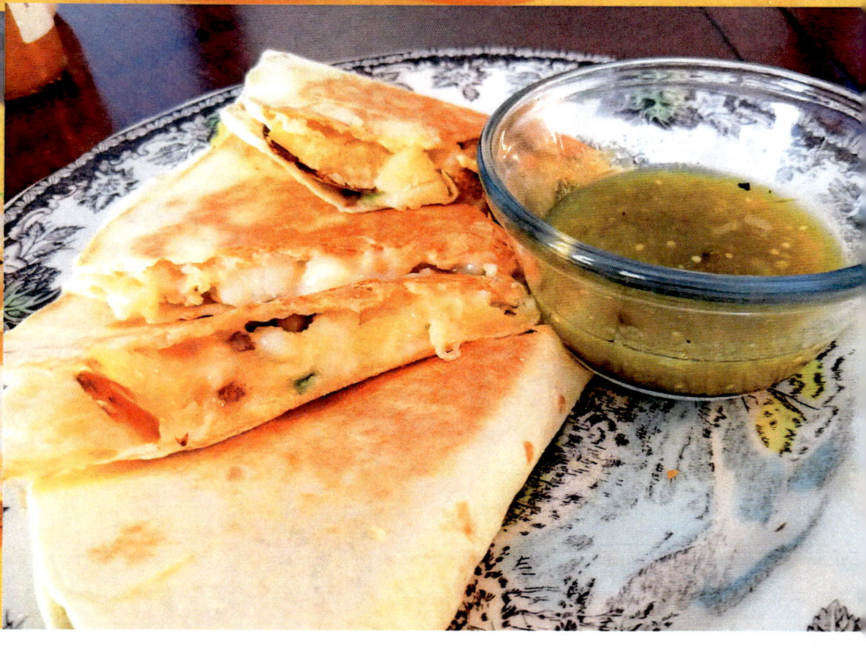

Radical Rice + Beans

serves 1-2

- 1 cup short or medium grain white rice
- 2 cups cold water
- 1 cup fresh greens (collards, kale, spinach, etc.)
- 1/2 green bell pepper, chopped (optional)
- Any kind of bean (black, kidney, pinto, etc.), rinsed (see page 11 for rinsing hack) -OR- black bean soup (1 15-ounce can)
- Salt and pepper to taste

In a large microwave safe bowl or container, combine rice and water. Loosely cover and microwave on high for 10 minutes. Check and if water has been absorbed and rice is fluffy, you're good to go. If not, microwave an additional minute.

Add greens, beans and salt and pepper to taste. (Optional: return to microwave for 30-60 seconds to steam greens.)

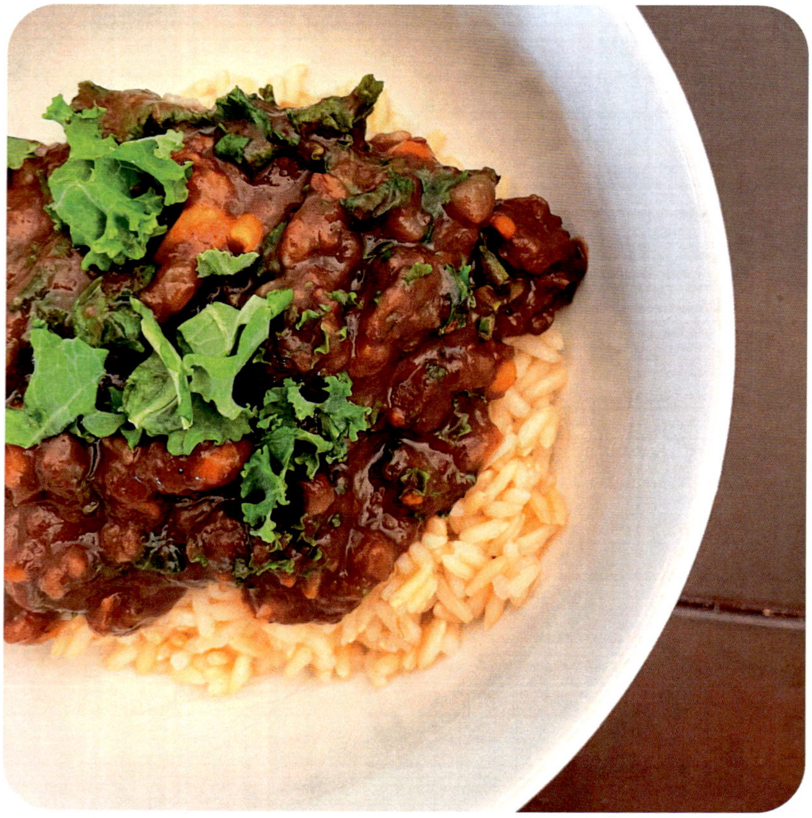

Salad Sandwich

serves 1

- 2 slices of your favorite bread (a darker or grainier bread is our favorite)
- 4-6 TBSP your favorite hummus
- 3-4 tomato slices
- 4-5 red onion slices, sliced very thinly
- 8-10 cucumber slices
- 1-2 slices vegan cheese (optional)
- Several pieces of your favorite lettuce (iceberg, arugula, romaine, butter, etc.)

Spread one side of each slice of bread with 2-3 TBSP hummus. Layer your veggies (and vegan cheese, if using) on one slice and place second slice on top. Cut in half diagonally (if you're feelin' snazzy) and dive in!

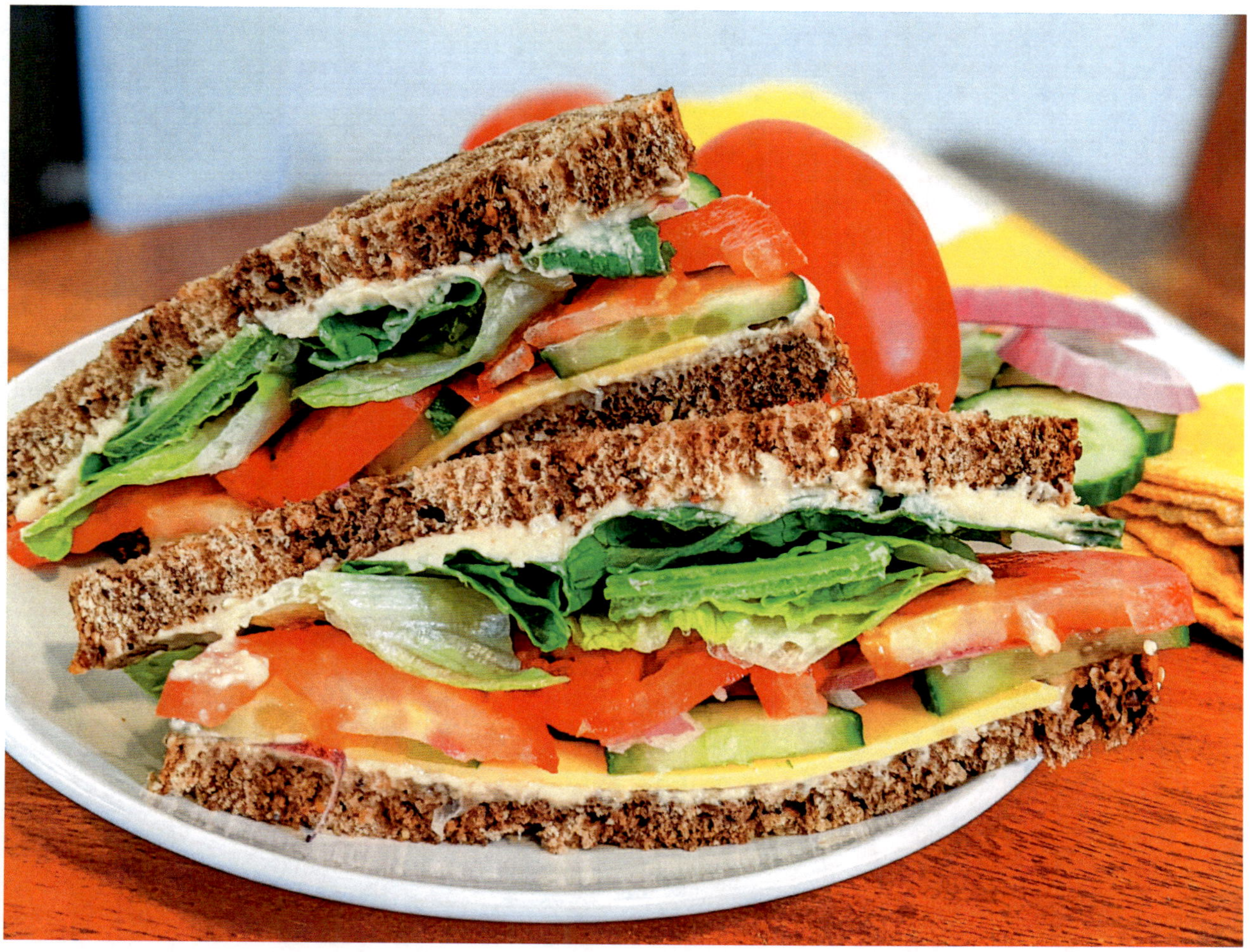

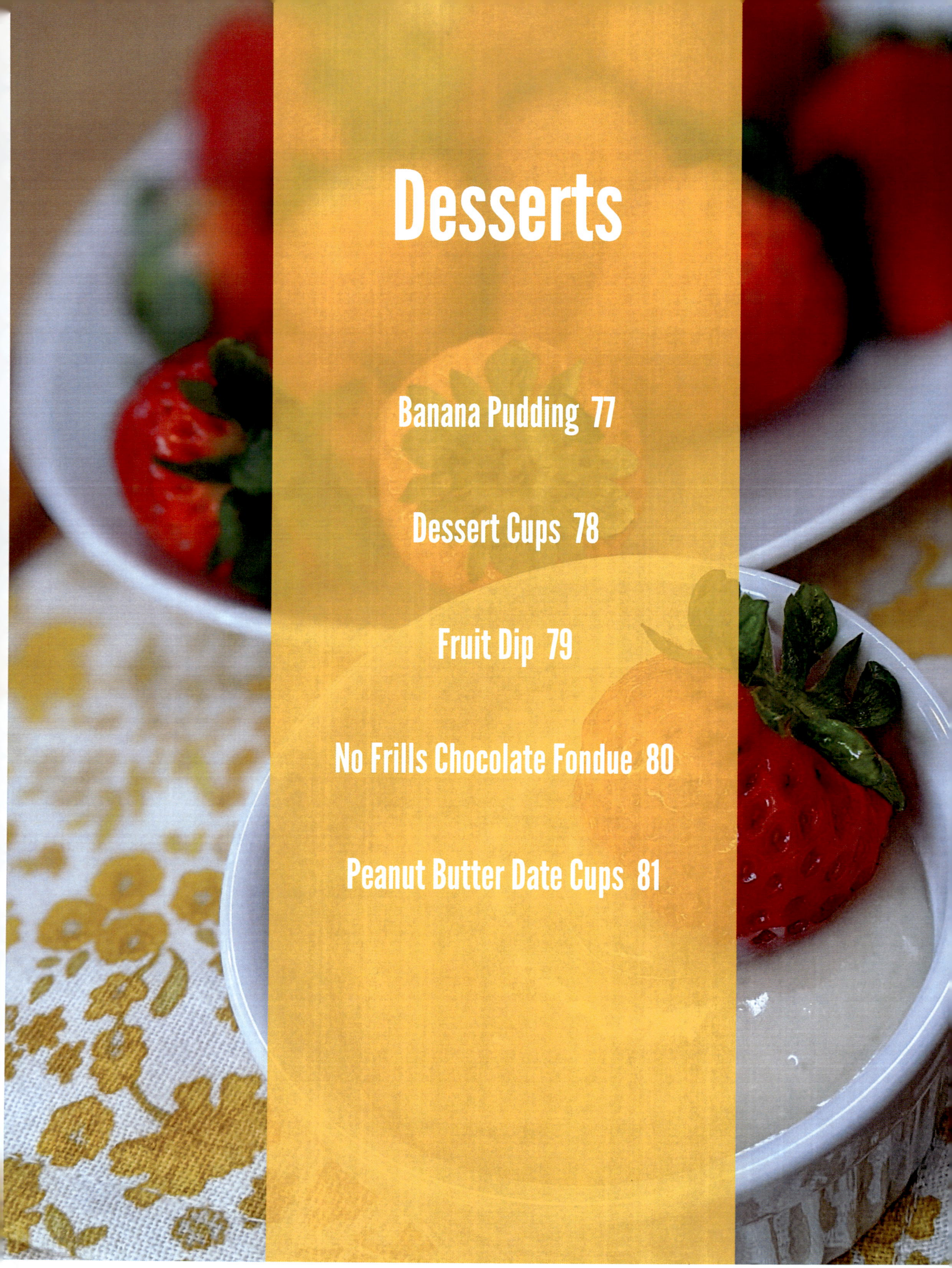

Desserts

Keeps well

Banana Pudding

2-4 depending on serving size

- 1 15-ounce can coconut milk (full-fat, unsweetened)
- 3 ripe bananas
- Cinnamon + salt (to taste)

Peel and mash all three bananas in a bowl. Open coconut milk can and scoop out the thick top layer of coconut cream (see notes). Add this cream to bowl of mashed bananas. Stir with a fork (or whisk if you have one). Add a sprinkle of cinnamon and a pinch of salt. Stir to combine.

The pudding will have a slight rice pudding texture with little bursts of coconut flavor and will keep well in the fridge for several days.

To serve: add fresh fruit, crumbled vanilla cookies, a scoop of non-dairy whip cream, and/or a handful of chopped peanuts.

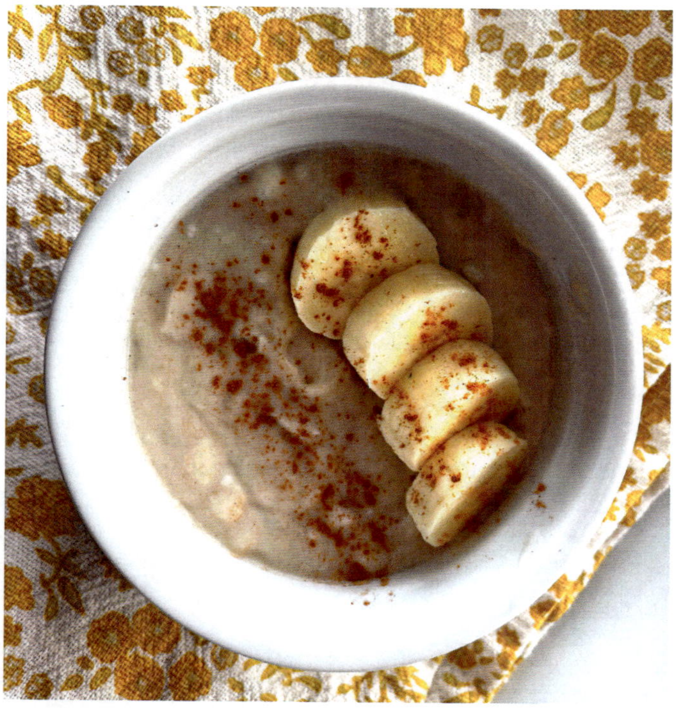

NOTES: You can use the leftover coconut milk liquid in our Oatmeal Bowls (page 64) or as the cooking liquid for our recipes that include rice!

Dessert Cups

Serves 1-2

PB+J Cup

- Mix 1/4 cup oats with a dash of cinnamon and 1 teaspoon maple syrup
- Use a fork to press oat mixture on bottom of bowl or container

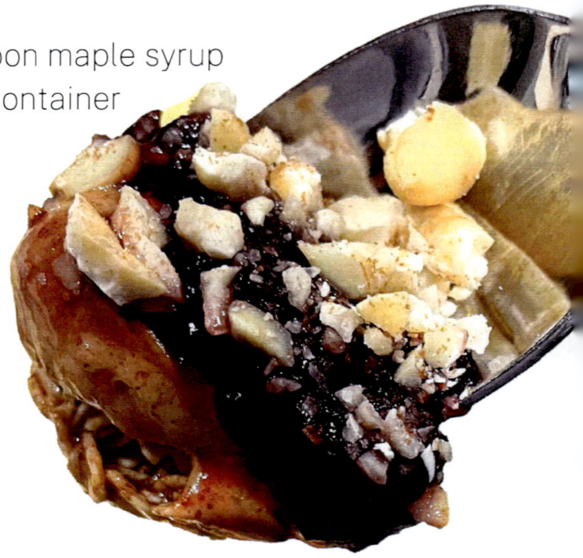

Layer on top:
- A thick layer of nut butter (we like crunchy almond)
- A medium-thick layer of jelly (your choice)
- A handful of crushed nuts (we like cashews)

Then:
- Place in the fridge for 1-2 hours
- Enjoy!

S'mores Cup

Dandies vegan marshmallows!

- Place a handful of cookies (vegan-friendly) in a Ziploc bag + smash with a spoon or your palm until you have crumbs
- Microwave 1 TBSP vegan butter until melted (20-30 seconds) + combine with cookie crumbs in a bowl - your "crust"
- Use a spoon to level this cookie crust along the bottom of bowl
- Add 1/4 cup vegan chocolate chips + 1 TBSP coconut oil (or vegan butter) to a separate bowl and microwave 30 seconds, stir
- Spread chocolate layer on top of cookie crumb layer
- Add crushed nuts, vegan marshmallows, and more cookie crumbs
- Enjoy!

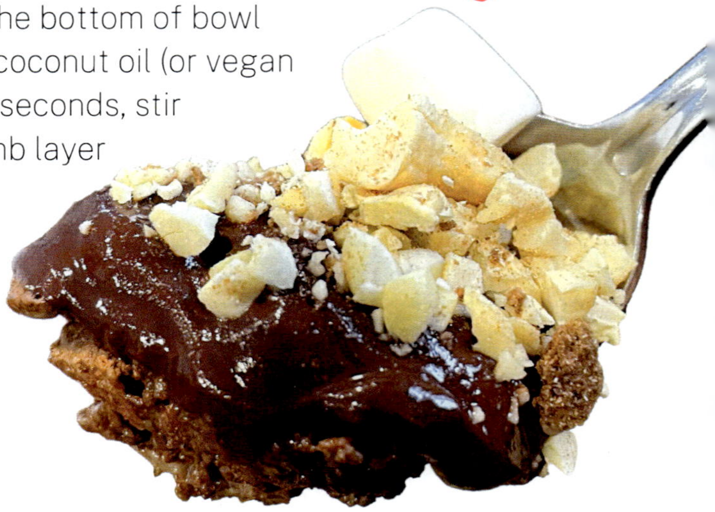

Fruit Dip

serves 1-2

- 1 pint strawberries, rinsed

DIP:

- 6 TBSP vegan cream cheese
- 2 TBSP maple syrup (see notes)
- 1/2 teaspoon vanilla (optional)

Place cream cheese in microwave safe dish and microwave for about 20 seconds or until softened. Add maple syrup (and vanilla, if using) and stir vigorously with a fork until well blended. Now you're ready to dip the strawberries in and enjoy!

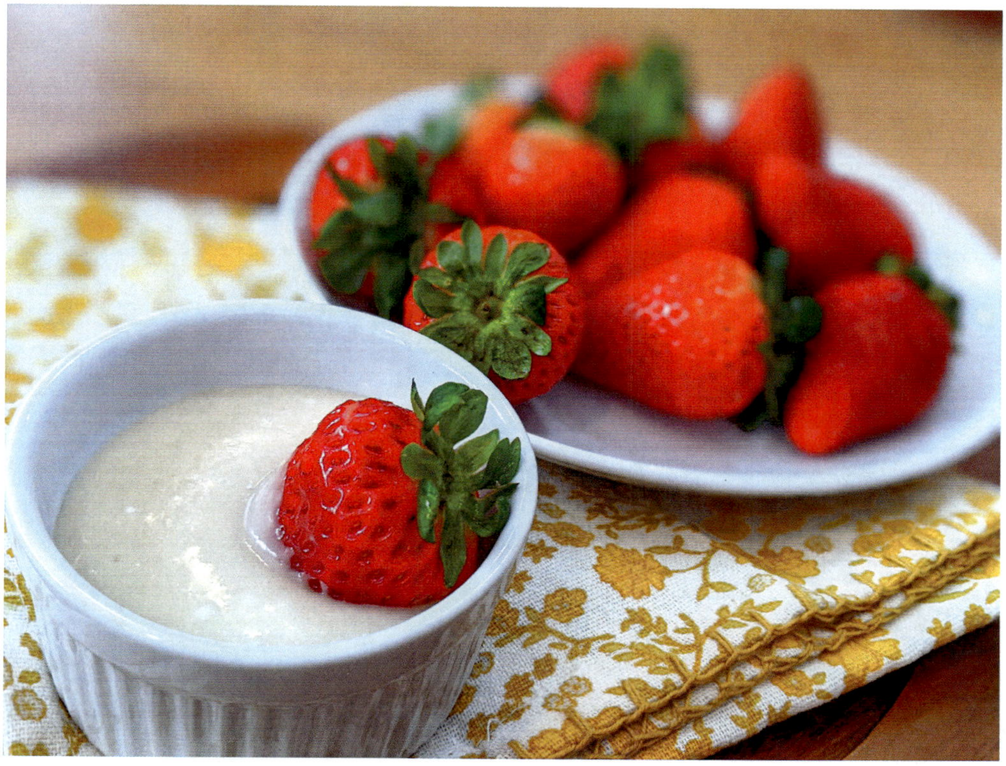

NOTES: You can use brown sugar for this recipe in place of maple syrup, but the result may be a bit grainy (unless you blend using beaters/handheld mixer). You can also try agave or another sweetener, but we can't vouch for the results!

No Frills Chocolate Fondue

serves 1-2

DIP:

- 1/3 cup semi-sweet, dairy-free chocolate chips (see notes)
- 2-3 TBSP coconut cream

DIPPERS:

- Vegan cookies (Oreos, Nutter Butters, Vanilla Wafers) and/or pretzels
- Fresh fruit

Place chocolate chips and coconut cream in microwave safe dish and microwave for about 20-30 seconds or until chocolate chips begin to soften. Stir with a spoon until chips continue to melt. You may need to microwave for a few seconds more, but be very careful not to burn chocolate!

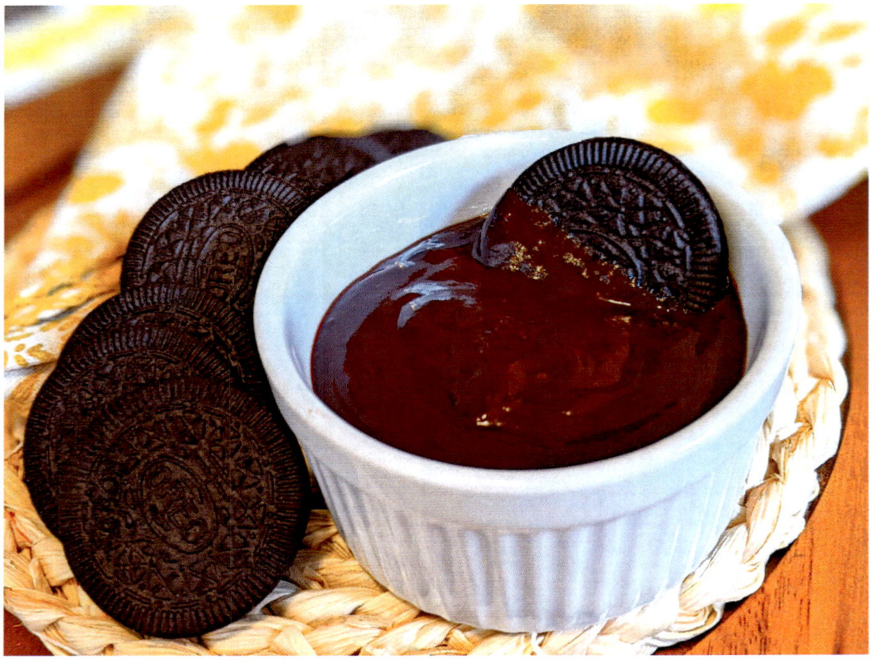

NOTES: Many name brand semi-sweet or dark chocolate chips are accidentally vegan and a lot cheaper than the 'dairy/allergy-free' brands. Just do a quick check of the bolded allergen section [on the ingredients label] for 'milk.'

Peanut Butter Date Cups

Keeps well

yields 24 “cups”

- 12 dates, sliced in half and pitted
- ½ cup peanut butter (see notes)
- ½ cup raisins
- Dash of cinnamon and salt

Scoop about ½ tablespoon peanut butter into the center of each pitted date half. Add a few raisins, a sprinkle of cinnamon, and dash of salt. Once your cups are assembled, refrigerate for at least one hour, then serve and enjoy!

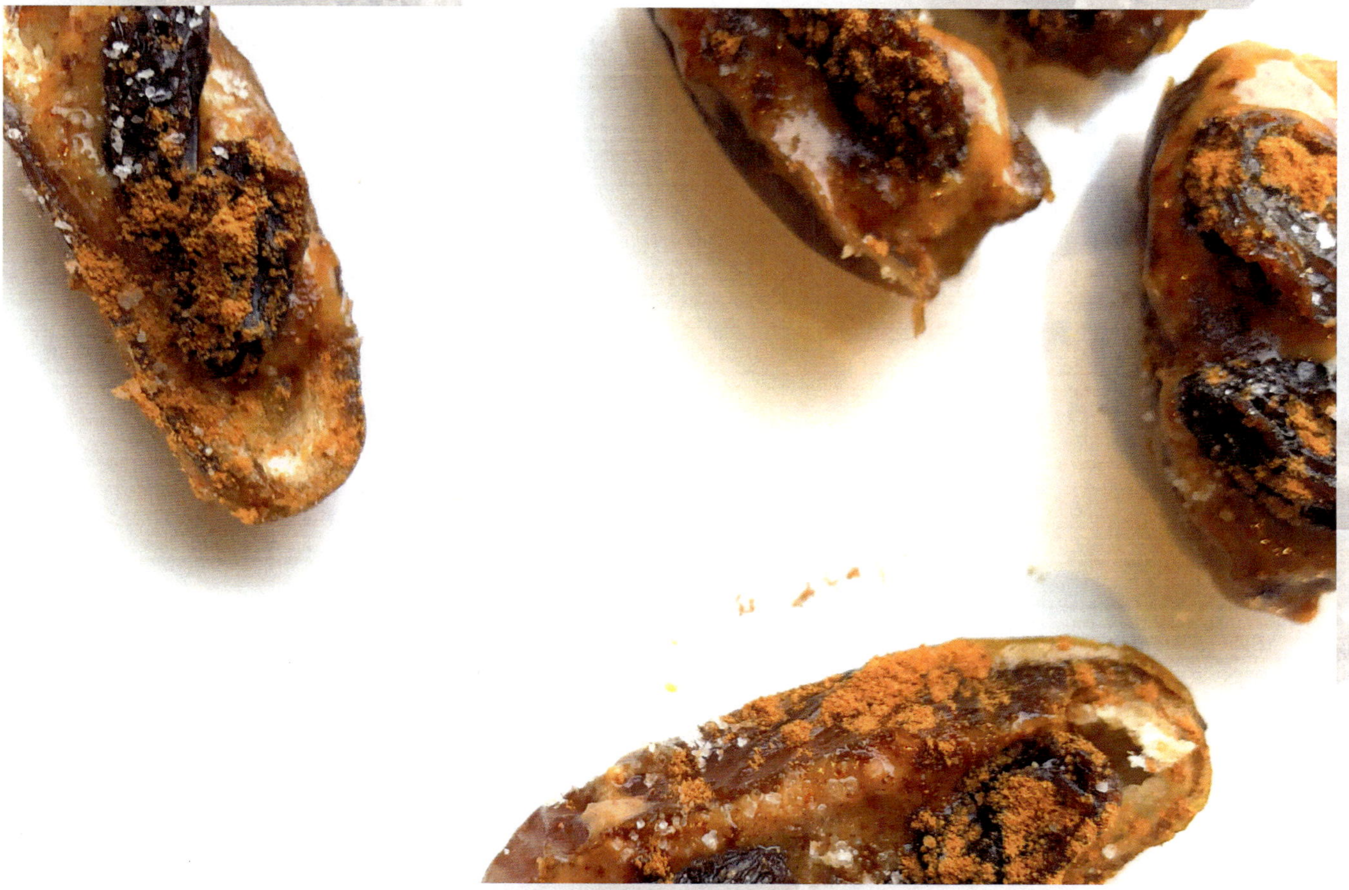

NOTES: These make a fantastic, healthy study snack to share and keep well in the fridge! You can swap out peanut butter with any nut or seed butter. You can also add crushed nuts, non-dairy chocolate chips, or whatever toppings sound good to you!

Store-Bought Wins

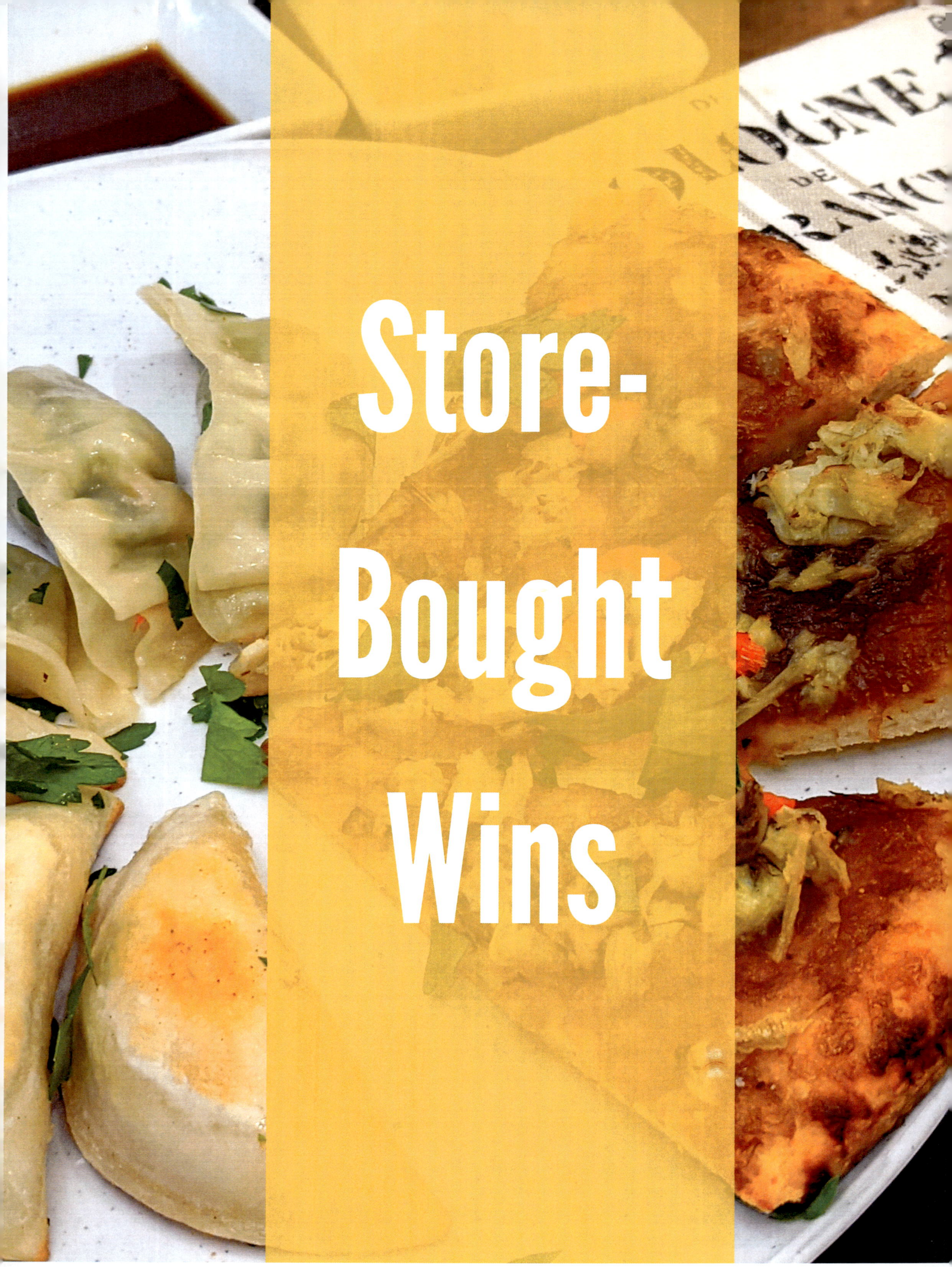

Appetizers

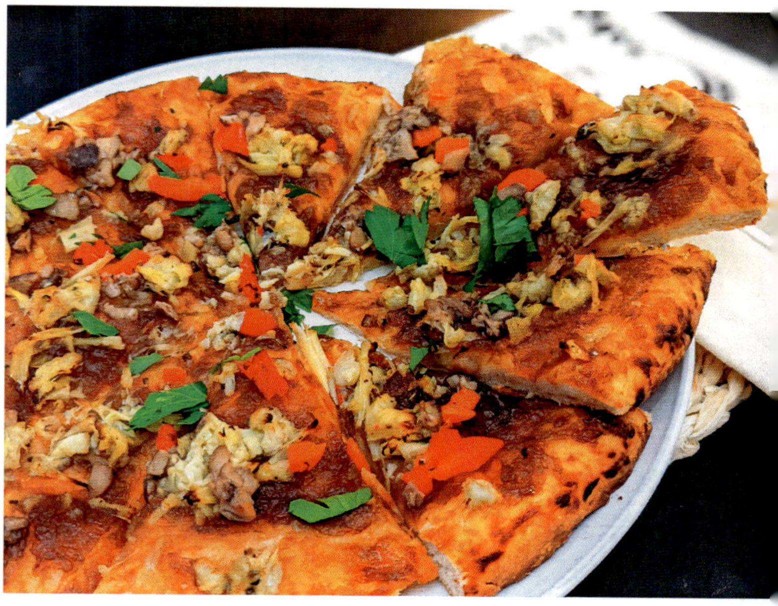

Frozen cheeseless (or vegan) pizza makes a fantastic appetizer and often goes on sale - simply slice into 8-12 slivers and serve!

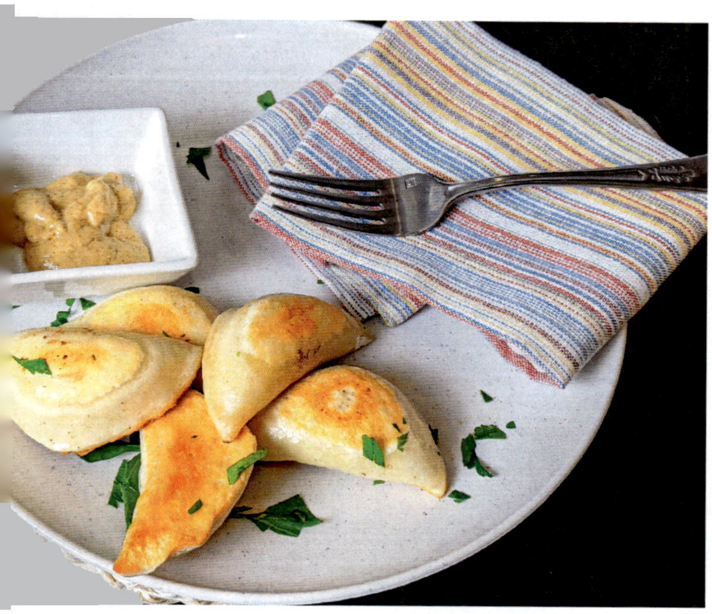

Potato + onion pierogis are usually accidentally vegan and dirt cheap! Serve with vegan sour cream and/or ketchup. Or, turn it into a meal by adding onions, greens, and vegan sausage!

Everyone we know loves a good veggie potsticker (gyoza) and they steam well in the microwave!

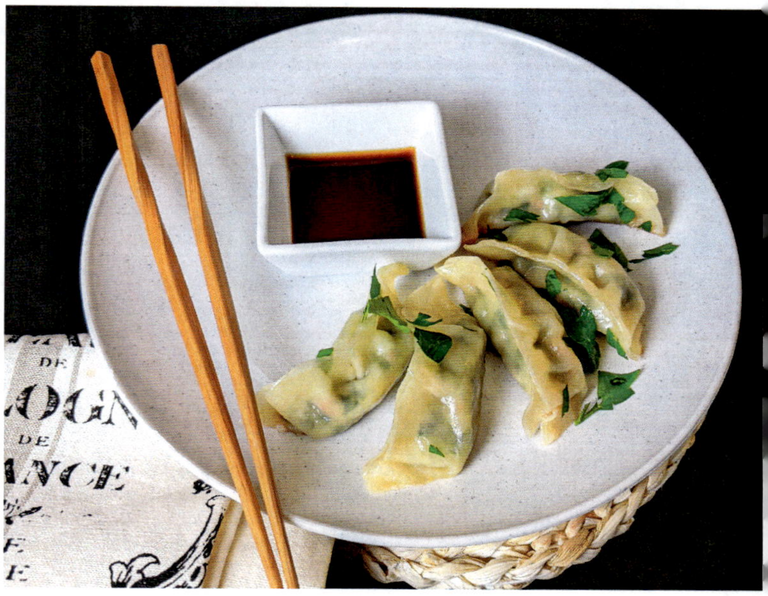

Mains

Buy a bag of frozen meatless balls and microwave with some of your favorite tomato sauce. (Toss on some pine nuts and/or parsley if you're feeling extra fancy.)

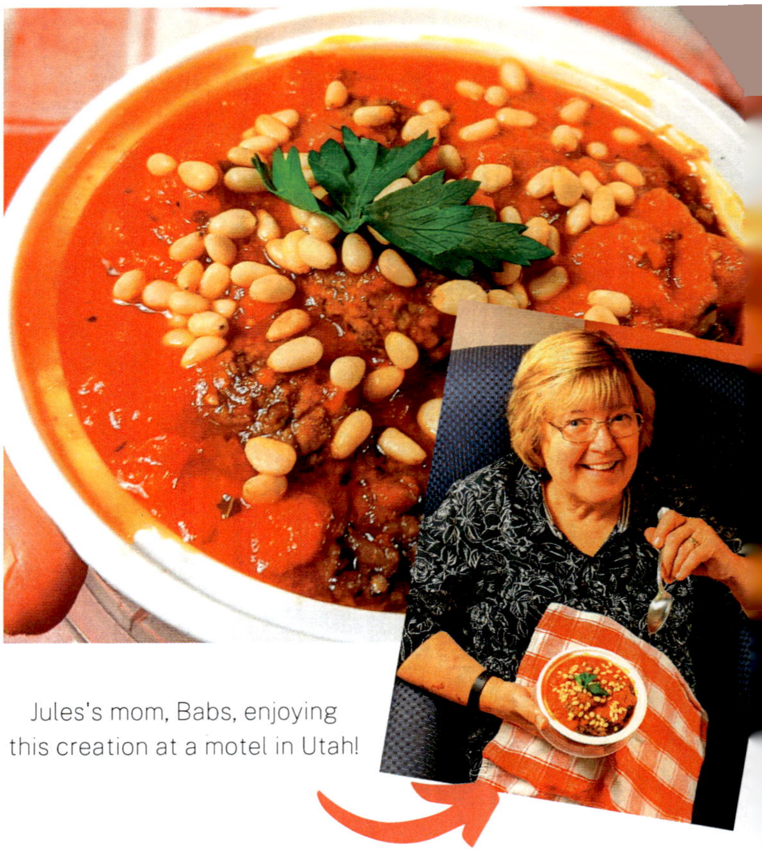

Jules's mom, Babs, enjoying this creation at a motel in Utah!

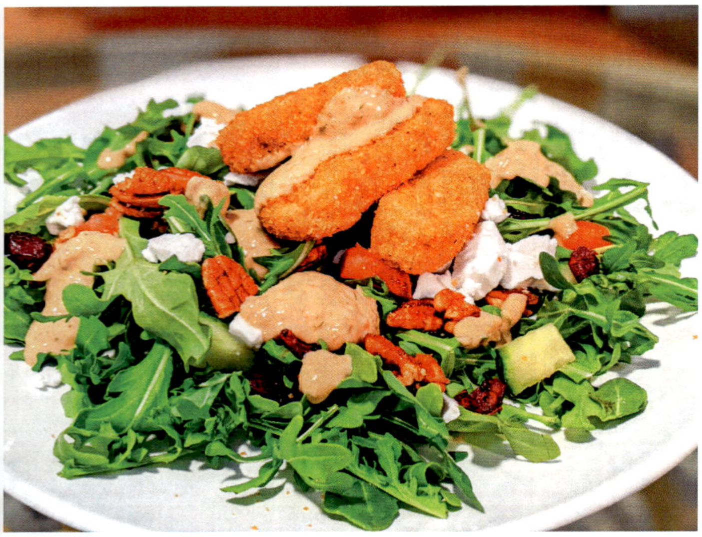

Frozen chick'n tenders make the perfect addition to any salad, quesadilla, panini, Italian dish, or pita pizza!

An easy win: most condiments are accidentally vegan, so grab a plant-based hot dog and go to town!

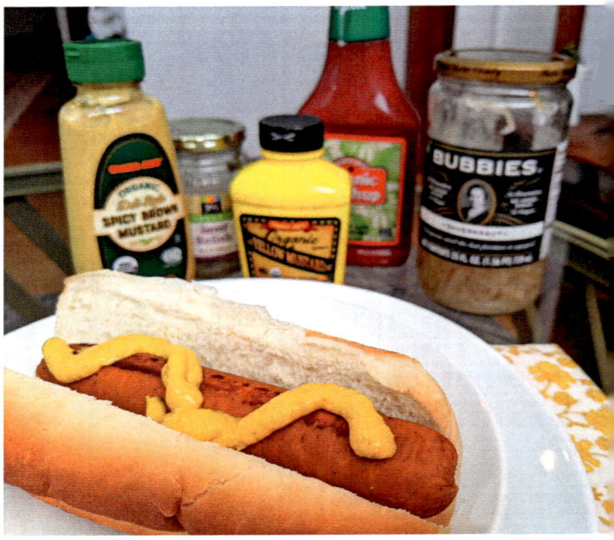

Desserts

The dairy-free ice cream, ice cream sandwich, and ice cream bar options are starting to overtake the non-vegan options - and we love them all! Even better, so many sundae toppings are accidentally vegan, too!

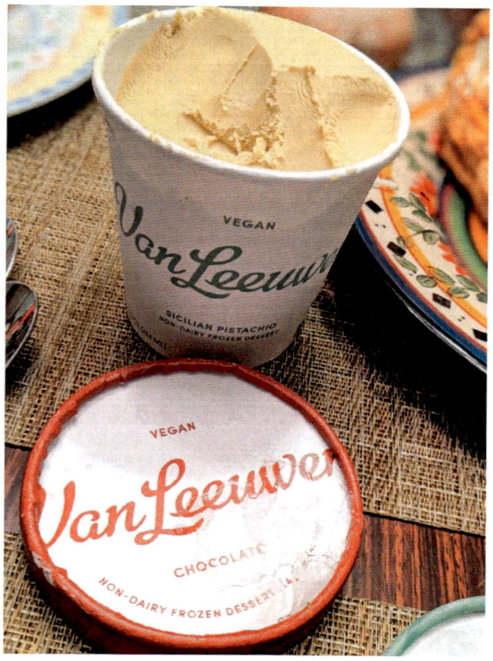

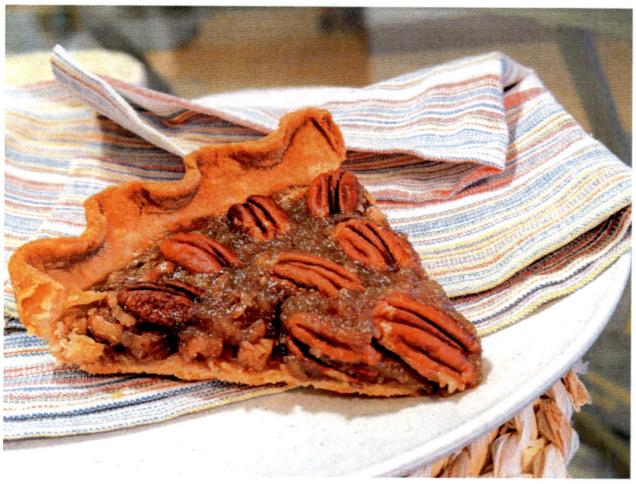

Many store-bought pie doughs and crusts, along with puff pastry, waffles, crescent rolls, and phyllo dough, are accidentally vegan and easily turned into epic desserts!

We've road tested many vegan butters, cream cheeses, sour creams, and egg substitutes and can vouch that most work perfectly in baked goods! Be sure to follow our YouTube channel for the latest taste tests and kitchen experiments!

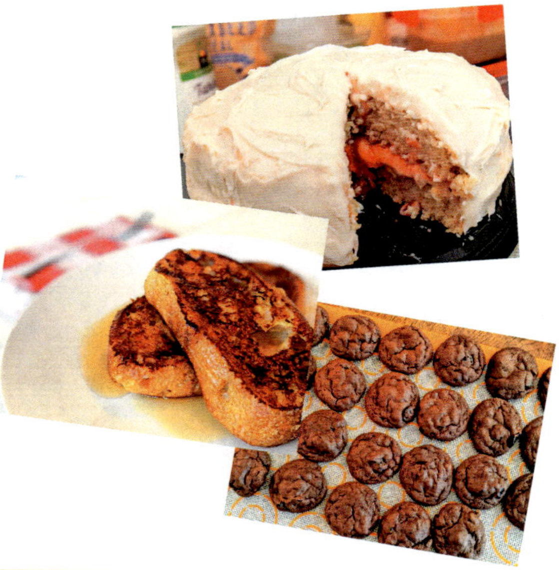

About the Authors

ROBIN COARTS

After years of eating vegetarian, Robin made the leap to vegan shortly after having her first son. Fast forward a few years, and a few compelling books and documentaries later, and she and her whole family (husband and two sons) are enjoying plant-based eating and living. Along the way, Robin started doing presentations at local libraries on the benefits of eating plant-based. After meeting Jules and discovering a shared sense of humor and commitment to education, Plant-Based Point launched.

Robin holds an M.S. in thanatology (Hood College), M.Ed in humane education (Institute for Humane Education + Valparaiso University), B.S. in gerontology, B.S. in psychology (both Towson University), and a Plant-Based Nutrition Certificate from eCornell. When she's not busy cooking, learning about, or talking all things plant-based, you'll find her running after two sons, spending time with her husband, or hitting the trails.

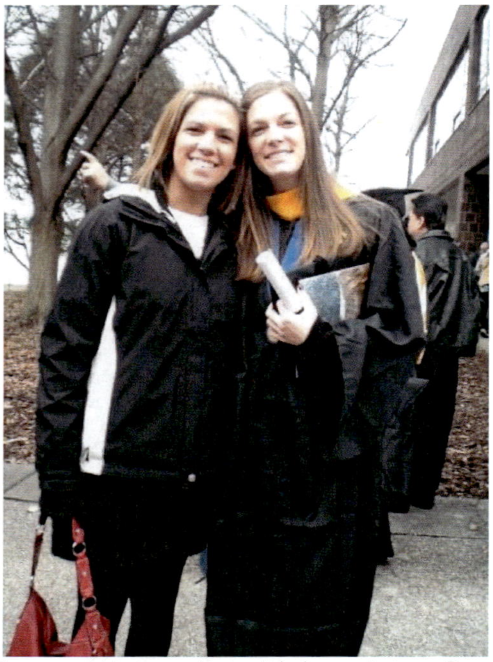

Towson University with her sister, Sara

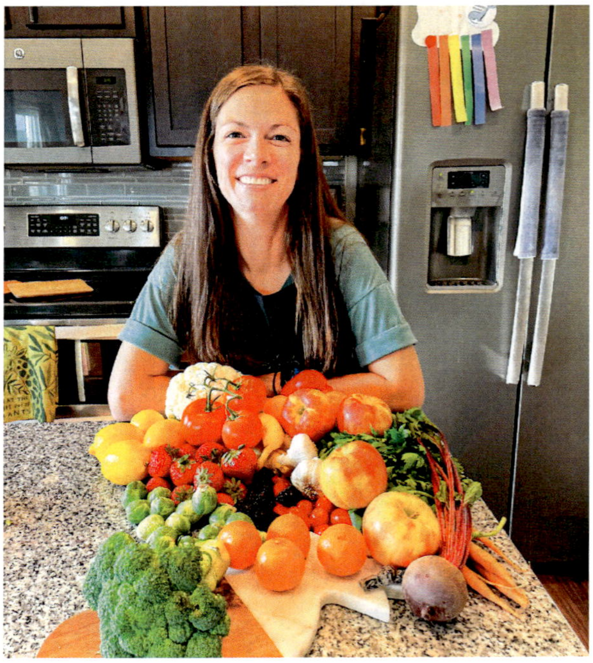

About the Authors

JULES SCHNEDEKER

Jules went vegan overnight in 2016 after watching the documentary, *Forks Over Knives*. She suddenly saw the impact our everyday food choices have on *everything*: the planet, non-human animals, and our health. In fact, this change was so transformative that Jules eventually quit her corporate job, moved across the country with nothing but her car and her dog, and put her money where her mouth was by co-founding Plant-Based Point.

Jules holds an M.A. in humane education (Institute for Humane Education + Valparaiso University), B.A. in creative writing (The New School), and a project management professional (PMP) certification. She's the author of the nonfiction humor blog, GoJulesGo.com, and when she's not busy telling her dog, Uncle Jesse, how cute he is, she's usually scouting new vegan products, trail running, or hiking the beautiful Oregon wilderness.

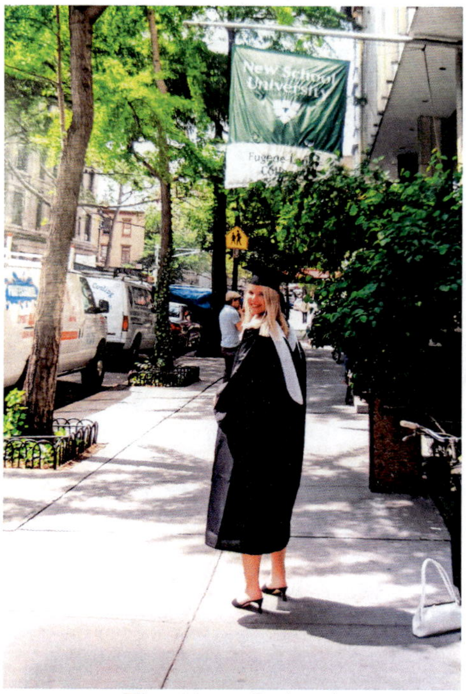

The New School

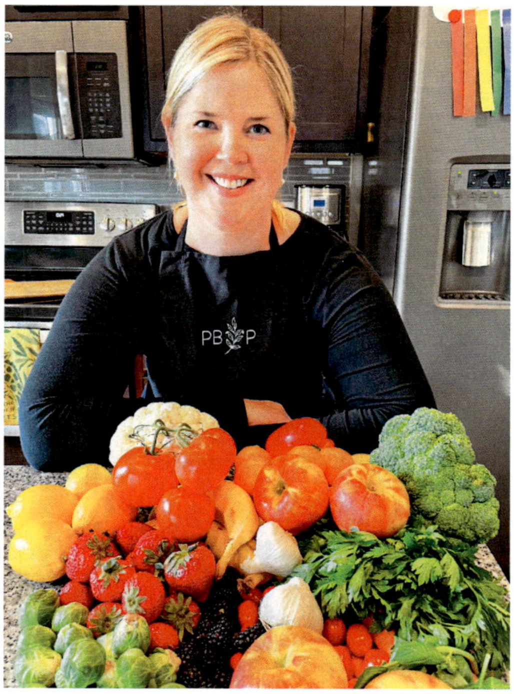

INDEX

Made in United States
North Haven, CT
13 November 2026

22102017R00051